Plague and Public Health in Early Modern Seville

Rochester Studies in Medical History

Senior Editor: Theodore M. Brown
Professor of History and Preventive Medicine
University of Rochester

ISSN 1526-2715

Additional Titles of Interest

Ludwik Hirszfeld: The Story of One Life
Edited by Marta A. Balińska and William H. Schneider
Translated by Marta A. Balińska

John W. Thompson: Psychiatrist in the Shadow of the Holocaust
Paul J. Weindling

*The Origins of Organ Transplantation:
Surgery and Laboratory Science, 1880–1930*
Thomas Schlich

Communities and Health Care: The Rochester, New York, Experiment
Sarah F. Liebschutz

The Neurological Patient in History
Edited by L. Stephen Jacyna and Stephen T. Casper

The Birth Control Clinic in a Marketplace World
Rose Holz

Bacteriology in British India: Laboratory Medicine and the Tropics
Pratik Chakrabarti

Barefoot Doctors and Western Medicine in China
Xiaoping Fang

Beriberi in Modern Japan: The Making of a National Disease
Alexander R. Bay

The Lobotomy Letters
Mical Raz

A complete list of titles in the Rochester Studies in Medical History series
may be found on our website, www.urpress.com.

Plague and Public Health in Early Modern Seville

KRISTY WILSON BOWERS

UNIVERSITY OF ROCHESTER PRESS

First published 2013

University of Rochester Press
668 Mt. Hope Avenue, Rochester, NY 14620, USA
www.urpress.com
and Boydell & Brewer Limited
PO Box 9, Woodbridge, Suffolk IP12 3DF, UK
www.boydellandbrewer.com

ISBN-13: 978-1-58046-451-2
ISSN: 1526-2715

Library of Congress Cataloging-in-Publication Data

Bowers, Kristy Wilson.
 Plague and public health in early modern Seville / Kristy Wilson Bowers.
   pages cm. — (Rochester studies in medical history ISSN 1526-2715 ; volume 26)
 Includes bibliographical references and index.
 ISBN 978-1-58046-451-2 (hardcover : alk. paper) 1. Plague—Spain—Seville—
History—16th century. 2. Plague—Prevention. 3. Medicine, Medieval—Spain—
Seville. I. Title.
 RC178.S72B69 2013
 616.9'2320094686—dc23

                                                    2013011380

A catalogue record for this title is available from the British Library.

This publication is printed on acid-free paper.
Printed in the United States of America.

To
Don E. Wilson and Kathleen Hayes Wilson,
with thanks for their continued
enthusiasm and encouragement.

Contents

Acknowledgments

Like many other academic studies, this work has been a remarkably long time in the making. When I first came across the extensive city council records of the sixteenth-century plague epidemics in Seville, I was little interested in matters of city governance or public health. Instead, I hoped to find similarly rich documents on the medical practitioners and practices within the city. Having found these records tucked away in different sections of the municipal archive, however, I began to read them for medical information and found myself increasingly drawn into the stories they told. Little did I realize that I would find myself working with them well over a decade later, still finding new details and new perspectives for analysis. Thus, my debts of support for both research and writing stretch back over many years. I owe first and foremost thanks to the mentors who most influenced my research: Helen Nader, who introduced me to early modern Spain, and Ann Carmichael, who introduced me to the history of plague. Both played pivotal roles in encouraging my early research and writing, and both influenced my subsequent intellectual development. I am enormously grateful for their support, encouragement, and guidance over many years.

Financial support for research trips at various stages has come from the Program for Cultural Cooperation Between Spain's Ministry of Culture and United States' Universities, the Society for the History of Pharmacy, the John C. Andressohn research fund at Indiana University, and the history department at Northern Illinois University. That funding has enabled my research at many institutions, and I am grateful for the assistance of many archivists and librarians. In Seville, I thank the archivists at the Archivo Municipal de Sevilla, the Archivo de la Diputación Provincial, the Archivo de Protocolos, and at the University of Seville. In addition, archivists in Simancas, Córdoba, Carmona, and especially in Loja helped me locate related records, many of which I could not have found on my own. The helpful staff at the National Library of Medicine was of great assistance in providing copies of many sixteenth-century treatises and texts.

In addition, I owe a great deal of thanks to many people over the years who have listened and responded to so many pieces of this work, far too many to mention individually. Nearly all the chapters began as conference papers presented at a variety of venues including the American Historical

Association, the Arizona Center for Medieval and Renaissance Studies, the American Association for the History of Medicine, the Association for Spanish and Portuguese Historical Studies, and the Sixteenth Century Society. In all these forums, I have been delighted by the interest and feedback given by colleagues in a variety of fields and have benefited greatly from collegial discussions.

My deepest thanks go to Valentina Tikoff, who has been a wonderful friend and colleague, and who has patiently listened to me talk about plague for far too many years, giving endless advice and support. Additional thanks to Michele Clouse, who has generously shared her own expertise on the medical world of sixteenth-century Spain, and to Beatrix Hoffman, who offered a critical eye to several chapters and much needed moral support. In addition, the anonymous readers of the manuscript offered comments that were both thoughtful and helpful, and I appreciate their assistance.

The underlying concept of "balance," as well as the arguments of chapters 3 and 4, were originally published as an article, "Balancing Individual and Communal Needs: Plague and Public Health in Early Modern Seville," *Bulletin of the History of Medicine* 81 (2007): 335–58. © 2007 by the Johns Hopkins University Press. I am grateful for permission to rework and expand those ideas here. Thanks also to Jodi Heitcamp and the Cartography Laboratory at Northern Illinois Univeristy for providing patient assistance in compiling the map of sixteenth-century towns.

My family has been enormously supportive all these years, and I am especially appreciative of the tireless support of my parents, Don and Kate Wilson. Finally, like all academics who constantly try to balance work and family, I give my love and thanks to J. D., Caroline, and Julia for always keeping me grounded in the present while I'm living in the past.

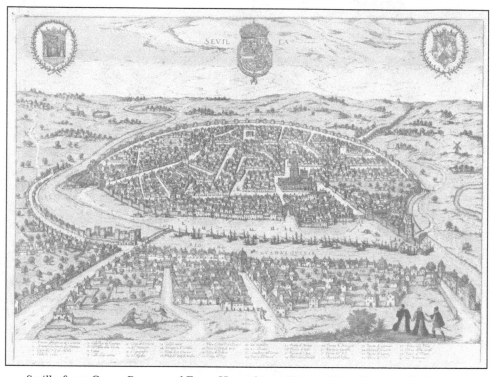

Sevilla, from Georg Braun and Frans Hogenberg, *Civitatis Orbis Terrarum* (Cologne, 1588), bk. 4. Courtesy of Princeton University Library, Department of Rare Books and Special Collections, Historic Maps Collection.

Introduction

The first half of the twentieth century brought the hope and expectation that modern science could eradicate disease, that humanity could dominate and control its greatest unseen enemy, microbes. In the 1940s new penicillin treatments helped reduce deaths from infections, while further advances in vaccines helped reduce or eradicate common childhood diseases such as measles, whooping cough, and smallpox. But the lessons of the second half of the century showed just how difficult true mastery of the microscopic world would be, as microbes continued to mutate, shift, and jump from one host to another. Emerging diseases, many of them transferred from animal hosts, such as Hantavirus, Ebola, and Avian Influenza, have continued to challenge medical researchers to find new ways of identifying and preventing such transfers.[1] Other emerging diseases such as Sudden Acute Respiratory Syndrome (SARS) and drug-resistant strains of tuberculosis (MDR-TB and XDR-TB) and staphylococcus (MRSA), combined with modern airline travel, have posed new problems to state authorities attempting to limit the spread of contagious diseases. These efforts have included restricting travel to or from certain areas, quarantining individuals (sometimes against their will), and the wholesale removal and slaughter of livestock, including chickens and pigs, in an attempt to prevent further spread of diseases despite the cost to individuals and communities.[2] All such efforts have prompted renewed debates about the power of the state to coerce individuals and the right of individuals to resist confinement. These debates are not new, however, and societies have long wrestled with questions of how best to prevent or reduce the spread of epidemics.[3]

Long before the term "emerging disease" had been coined, there were the "pestilential" epidemics of the early modern era. These were the years now often identified as the second pandemic of plague, in which epidemics disrupted lives and routines across Europe, beginning with the vast and deadly pandemic now commonly known as the Black Death (1347–52), which continued to recur in local epidemics into the eighteenth century.[4] Seen as emerging from a variety of causes including weather, environment, miasmas, and poor diet, these pestilential epidemics prompted lengthy medical debates over health, disease, and the most effective means of both prevention and treatment. In the century following the Black Death, ideas of

.tagion emerged with new force alongside ideas of environmental causes
disease, among both civic leaders and physicians.[5] Yet the ideas of conta-
zion that emerged in this time period were varying and debated, as was the
diagnosis of pestilence itself. In the early modern era, diagnosis depended
on reading and interpreting symptoms, a practice that was neither simple
nor straightforward, but which required the knowledge, experience, and
skills of a trained medical practitioner—or so many of them claimed.

Early modern Europe embraced a range of these practitioners, from
university-educated physicians through apprentice-trained surgeons down
to the more lowly apothecaries and barber-surgeons. There were also, of
course, the less regulated practitioners: empirics, itinerants, faith healers,
and specialists who pulled teeth, punched cataracts, or removed anal fistula.
All of these practitioners played a crucial role in epidemics, offering a range
of treatments to the sick and convalescent. It was the regular practitioners—
physicians, surgeons, and apothecaries—who often also played a civic role
as consultants for city officials trying to monitor and manage epidemics.
Early modern public health efforts tend to look rather different from modern efforts; they appear chaotic at times and based more on personalities
than science. Yet when examined in context, these public health efforts hold
their own logic and accurately reflect the complex set of beliefs about health
of the premodern era.

This book examines public health as it was practiced—created, implemented, and revised—by city officials in late sixteenth-century Seville, particularly in response to epidemics identified as plague. Public health was a
chronic issue in the early modern era, periodically made critical by epidemic
waves of disease that port cities like Seville faced regularly. Physicians in the
sixteenth century attached specific diagnoses to these epidemics: cattarh
(*catarro*), typhus (*tabardete, tabardillo*), and plague (*peste, mal de peste*) were
common. But they also often used nonspecific terms, such as "pestilence"
(*enfermedad pestilencial*) or "contagion" (*mal contagioso*), terms that took on
different shades of meaning at different times. Whatever the terminology
used, officials knew well the toll that these epidemics took not only in mortality within their cities, but also in economic depressions caused by a combination of high mortality and stringent quarantine measures that disrupted
the movement of both goods and people. As these epidemics continued over
centuries, officials gradually created subtle changes in the public health system in an effort to balance competing needs of public health against the
needs of economic and social stability.

For Seville, the records are too scarce from the early part of the century
to be able to pinpoint when this shift started. But the results come into sharp
focus by 1582, when the city's records clearly show new efforts to balance
competing demands. Officials in Seville, like many others across Europe,
responded to epidemics with what seems to us a strange balance of fear and

disregard. They imposed regulations, then allowed frequent exceptions; they banned travelers they feared might bring disease with them, then sent their own colleagues traveling to the very areas where disease was reported and allowed them to return to the city unimpeded. They asked physicians and surgeons for professional advice and then, often as not, chose to act against that advice. These and other seeming contradictions appear much more sensible when viewed through the lens of the era. Diseases, especially plague, were fluid and unpredictable; medicine, while rational and useful, was often of limited use in the face of God's will, environmental conditions, and social imbalances. By the sixteenth century, city officials had come to accept the continual threat of epidemics, whether of plague or other causes, and had gradually worked out new routines for how to deal with the questions, complaints, and uncertainties they brought. This then, is the focus of the book: how one early modern city adapted to living with periodic outbreaks of plague by developing new means to balance a variety of causative theories (miasmas, contagion, and diet), competing interests (medical and economic), and overlapping power structures (local and state officials).

Early Modern Plague

The ability of historians, microbiologists, or epidemiologists to definitively determine the cause of disease in the past is still often debated.[6] Retrospective diagnosis of either epidemics or of individual cases must often rest in interpreting the symptoms reported in various records. The greatest problem, of course, is that many of these records were not written for medical purposes, and even those written by physicians reflect the very different mindset of the pre–germ theory era. Currently, disease is identified by locating microscopic pathogens in the laboratory; many argue that it is impossible to assert with certainty what caused a described set of symptoms in the past without that microscopic verification. A description of fever, rash, headache, and loss of appetite, for example, could reasonably be attributed to measles, smallpox, or typhus. Recent and ongoing collaborative work between historians and microbiologists, aided by technological advances in extracting and analyzing DNA from bones and teeth, has helped provoke a reassessment of these questions of retrospective diagnosis, in an ongoing dialogue among experts in various fields.[7]

Among past epidemics, the cause of early modern "pestilence" has often been among the most contested in its identification. Arguments over how to identify these epidemics began in the 1990s and have continued sporadically in the decades since.[8] Very recent and ongoing work by microbiologists has now found evidence of *Yersinia pestis*, the causative agent of bubonic plague, in late medieval remains, leading to an ongoing reassessment among historians and epidemiologists.[9] Yet even while some historians have disputed the diagnosis of plague, many others have accepted the lack of clear specific diagnosis, focusing instead on the reported experiences and beliefs of people. For what remains undisputed is that early modern Europeans suffered epidemics that took a high toll in mortality and profoundly affected a variety of social, cultural, and economic patterns.

For many studies, including this one, what matters is not a modern diagnosis, but how people's experiences with disease shaped their societies. In order to understand these experiences, we must accept the mindset of the sixteenth century and remember that while physicians and city officials often used terms such as "plague" and "typhus" in ways that sound familiar, their understanding of those terms was quite different from ours. In the early modern world, disease was a fluid concept, and terms including "plague," "pest," and "pestilence" were both broad and flexible in their application. As discussed in detail in chapter 2, disease could even be identified by physicians as pestilential either in a dangerous sense or in an ordinary sense. Just as we today use the word "plague" as both a specific identifier for disease and as a general term to connote any feared epidemic, so did early modern writers use their terms loosely. As nineteenth-century scientists carried these terms forward and refined their definition through laboratory science, the names for diseases have become attached to very specific causes and very specific sets of symptoms.[10] Thus, adopting premodern terms to modern diagnoses has helped create an illusion of parallel experience between the premodern and modern eras that is too often false or impossible to verify. But the terms themselves are difficult to move away from—records from both medical and civic authorities are filled with them. Thus, when this work mentions plague, typhus, or other specific diseases, it does so as a reflection of the terms used in the sixteenth century. Where it seems helpful to do so, I have included in parentheses the exact words or phrases from the documents to help demonstrate this fluidity.

Plague in Historical Context

Studies of plague have traditionally focused attention on two aspects. The first is the dramatic and terrifying aspect of the Black Death, while the second is the development of medical response in the century following the Black Death. The first aspect of plague that is emphasized, and still the most often cited characteristic, is that of plague as a disruptive historical factor, creating chaotic breakdown that continued in repeated cycles over the four hundred years traditionally associated with the second pandemic of plague (1350–1720). Ranging from classic studies to recent popular histories, these works all emphasize both the newness and awfulness of plague, particularly during the fourteenth century.[11] Relying most often on the vivid firsthand descriptions of writers such as Giovanni Boccaccio and Gabriele de' Mussis, these works offer readers a clear image of fear and desperation. As de' Mussis recounts, "All have been destroyed; thrust aside by death. To whom shall we turn, who can help us? To flee is impossible, to hide futile."[12] Philip Ziegler's study of the Black Death written in the 1960s, though now clearly outdated, still nicely embodies this dramatic approach, asserting that "in the Middle Ages the plague was not only all-destroying, it was totally incomprehensible. Medieval man was equipped with no form of defense—social, medical or psychological—against a violent epidemic of this magnitude."[13] More recently, Joseph Byrne summarized daily life by asserting that "in plague time, this 'daily life' was suspended for virtually everyone. For some it meant abandoning everything and fleeing to a safe place, for others shutting themselves up in their homes to wait the epidemic out. . . . In cities, schools let out, churches closed, shops were abandoned, neighbors moved . . . the streets emptied of crowds."[14] Such descriptive works offer an image of one important aspect of plague, though many authors, it should be noted, also acknowledge that life did indeed go on despite plague. But the appeal of these works continues to lie in the drama and trauma that they present.

The second common focus of plague studies, especially in those more often written by medical historians, emphasizes the ways that this "new" disease helped lay the groundwork for modern concepts and practices, especially those of contagion and the subsequent development of quarantine and boards of health.[15] In these studies, officials in many Italian city-states, even if misguided in their understanding of why such measures were helpful, nonetheless foreshadowed modern isolation practices, though their efforts are often seen as of little use against an unenlightened population that often worked to circumvent these practices.[16]

That European civilization survived these epidemics, while still being changed by them, is clear. Many studies have demonstrated the acceptance of plague as part of life in the Renaissance, unwelcome though it may have been. Paul Slack's work on England shows that by the sixteenth century the crown had begun taking control of epidemic response, and while such measures were still met with resistance, there was what he terms "compromise" over them.[17] Likewise, William Naphy's study of plague-spreading conspiracies in Geneva, though focused primarily on accusations and trials of accused conspirators, offers a portrait of a sixteenth-century city with clear public health routines that enabled a measured response to epidemics, so that, he argues, "the citizenry felt that they had the tools and methods necessary for coping with, and ultimately surviving, the epidemic."[18]

The present study continues this mode of analysis, using the idea of balance as the best means to understand the complex ways that epidemics affected lives and people responded. It shows that rather than continuing to respond to plague with just the fear and panic shown in the fourteenth century, people adjusted to living with plague epidemics and worked out routines of response that enabled trade and travel to continue (albeit at a modified pace). What enabled this continuity was not "modernity" as heralded by either a standing health board or new ideas of contagion. Instead, new concepts of contagion merged into miasmatic theory, creating entirely new and more complex concepts of the ways that disease did or did not pose dangers to the community or to individuals. These new concepts were embraced in differing ways by city officials and medical authorities, which led to an equally complex system of public health. While these concepts seem at times incongruous or inconsistent within our current framework for health and disease, they reveal the strikingly different mindset of early modern culture, which predicated disease on a multiplicity of factors. Mixed into this framework also, we must remember, were very different concepts of locality, class, and status that additionally colored beliefs on who or what could be polluting to the environment or individual. Thus, while early modern plague epidemics certainly affected all levels of society and produced profound changes in urban routines, they also became one more aspect of life needing to be balanced with all others.

A large part of the new balances worked out in public health were a result of the understanding of disease in the early modern era. The Galenic system developed in the ancient world was still unchallenged in the early modern one. Flexible in its diagnosis, treatment, and preventive regimens, Galenic humoralism continually adapted to different symptoms and outcomes, providing a broad theoretical framework that embraced ideas of change and fluidity. Look into any aspect of the history of medicine in this era and you will find a plethora of types of practitioners, types of training, and treatment regimens. While all agreed that humoral theory dictated the development of symptoms, there was often disagreement on how best to interpret or apply humoral theory in individual cases. Even royal families retained a number of physicians, in part because different practitioners held different expertise, but in part so that if the treatments of one seemed ineffective, others could be consulted instead. Thus, there was rarely a single answer to the question of whether or not a pestilential epidemic was present in communities—it could be both yes and no, depending on who was asked. The question was a crucial one for city administrators, however, for experience had taught them to fear any illness that could spread rapidly through the population. In order to best contain the spread of pestilential epidemics, officials relied on separation: using quarantine to separate sick from healthy or keeping individuals dispersed by forbidding public gatherings. Such measures, however, often led to rebellion by citizens, which thwarted official efforts.[19] Keeping the population content (or at least preventing chaotic rebellion against authority) meant placating both sides, balancing conflicting views of how to define health and how best to maintain it.

While the early modern fight against plague did not create the earliest ideas of contagion, it should still be seen as ushering in an unexpectedly modern public health dilemma: the tensions between the rights of the community to be protected from those who pose a risk of spreading disease and the rights of individuals to live and travel without undue constraints on them. The term "rights" was not used in this era, and indeed the idea of individuals having rights would not fully emerge into the political lexicon, let alone into common understanding of the public, until much later. The modern public health dilemma of conflicting rights emerged most fully in the nineteenth century, but the need to find balance between individual and communal interests may certainly be traced back to the earliest public health regulations created in response to plague.[20]

Plague in Seville

Seville, like other Spanish cities, was governed by a city council. Councilmen juggled a variety of duties such as overseeing the collection of taxes and dues, regulating markets, contracting public works projects, and managing a variety of crises including epidemics, droughts, locust infestations, and food shortages. In order to do so, they sometimes appointed commissions or committees whose purpose was to oversee the management of specific issues. Among these were the health commissions, appointed from among councilmen when an epidemic spread. While they often consulted with physicians and surgeons, the commissions primarily monitored the number of sick and issued response legislation in an effort to limit the impact of crises.

One important function of the health commission was to investigate and collect information that could be used to make its decisions. These men knew all too well the disruption plague and plague regulations could cause. The commission collected and maintained extensive records related to epidemics, most of it recorded in tremendous detail including names, places, and dates within the *cuadernos de la peste*. But despite the detail in these notebooks, the records remain fragmentary and sporadic. Full notebooks have not survived for any epidemic, and those partial notebooks that do remain reflect a certain amount of discontinuity. Much of the work of the commission involved investigating what it termed "suspicious" illnesses, either within the city itself or in the towns of the *tierra*, to determine whether a dangerous epidemic could develop. But these investigations were often cursory, with little effort made to follow up or monitor cases after the initial contact. With the exception of some towns that maintained ongoing negotiations with the city council regarding their health status, the health commission's records present the beginnings of countless stories with few satisfactory endings. Instead, they offer glimpses into the lives of various residents and fragmentary stories that reflect the coping strategies of the city during epidemics. In part, the incomplete nature of these stories reflects the reason this information was collected in the first place. Nowhere in the records is there any attempt to lay blame or trace out the origins of the contagion; commissioners rarely followed up after a diagnosis of plague, for example, by tracing routes of exposure or contact between residents. Instead, the records reflect an effort to gain a sense of control. Councilmen were accustomed to keeping extensive notes on all their actions, and times of plague were no exception, as they made every effort to maintain standards and to approach epidemics rationally. At the same time, councilmen kept residents aware of their presence through continual investigations, asserting both a calming and supervisory presence by being visible in the streets. Thus, they worked to gain their own sense of control by gaining as much information as possible, while also maintaining public perception of their control over impending crises. The records therefore remain cursory because their purpose was not to create a narrative but rather to offer evidence of official efforts. They are in a sense snapshots of information that reflect the health commission's concerns regarding the emerging epidemic.

This kind of ad hoc response to epidemics, despite being rather widespread throughout many European cities, has received little attention and even less credit from historians. Instead, the much more formalized response that developed in several Italian city-states, emphasizing reliance on standing boards of health, represents the best-known model of early modern public health and is often referred to as the most advanced system then available.[21] In part, perhaps, these boards generated clearer records of their activities than those of temporary commissions whose records were often mixed into other city records. The result has been to relegate these temporary commissions to a secondary, less-effective status, or at least a less progressive one. Thus, William Naphy, after detailing the cool and measured response of Geneva's city council when epidemics appeared, nonetheless "raises the question of the lack of any permanent Health Board in the city," defending the city's *lack* by pointing to the work of the city's senate in closely overseeing these matters rather than delegating them.[22] Such defensiveness is unnecessary, however, as each system reflected different approaches and objectives. From a modern, materialist perspective, the Italian model of health boards may well have offered more effective disease control. If, however, we redefine public health more broadly, to include the notion of the overall well-being of the community, then the more flexible approach exemplified by the Genevan senate and the city council in Seville was quite successful. Rather than provoke resistance and unrest, Seville's city council worked to keep residents cooperative or at least compliant.

Historians have lauded the Italian regimen as forward-thinking, both because it set what would become the standard for all of Europe and because it may have had positive effects, despite lacking a modern understanding of disease transmission. Above all, the creation of permanent health boards is seen as a positive step in focusing the attention of civic leaders on public health. While some areas outside of Italy, particularly Aragon, created permanent health boards, most opted instead for temporary commissions, often composed principally of civic leaders who may have consulted with medical personnel at times. The larger difference, though, between Italian city-states and other European cities, such as Seville, may be found in the policies of these groups and how they enforced their regulations.

Civic leaders in the Italian city-states based their policies of exclusion as much on politics as public health. The proximity of small separate states in northern Italy made it both expedient and easy to simply exclude residents from neighboring cities in times of crisis. While in many cases these city-states held important economic ties, their separate political identities enabled them to more justifiably identify and exclude outsiders than was the case in most other European states. In Seville, for example, the ability of city leaders to exclude residents from nearby towns was limited, both because many such towns were part of Seville's political domain (whose residents therefore had certain rights clearly specified in the city's regulations, particularly of access to the municipal government) and because of the heavy economic and social interdependence between them. Even more distant cities that held no direct political ties to Seville, such as Granada or Córdoba, were not viewed by municipal officials with the same political antagonism as that found between, for example, the independent city-states of Florence and Milan.[23]

A second important difference is that in Italian cities, health boards were created as permanent entities, charged with continuously monitoring the city's residents even when epidemics were not imminent. Headed most often by nobles, boards were appointed for terms of varying length.[24] While they were often assisted or advised by physicians, these men were the principal administrators of public health policy and plague prevention, which was not a job to be taken lightly. Thus, those nobles placed in charge of monitoring public health, watching for signs of the next big eruption of plague, would naturally have been entirely focused on their task at hand. Their reputations depended on their diligence in carrying out those duties. Strict and uniform enforcement of plague regulations resulted as health commissioners sought to carry out their duties as carefully as possible.

The impact of this strict enforcement has been examined by a number of historians. Ann Carmichael and Brian Pullan have shown how plague regulations could shift into social control as definitions of at-risk populations increasingly focused on the poorer residents unable to flee the city.[25] Carlo

Cipolla's studies all emphasize the conflicts surrounding the enforcement of restrictions that arose between officials (particularly health officials) and residents. In acknowledging the difficult tasks facing health officers of the sixteenth century, for example, he argues that they "must have constantly experienced feelings of frustration as they watched their ordinances being obstructed by poverty, ignorance, stupidity, and vested interests."[26] Likewise, his study *Faith, Reason, and the Plague*, which examines the plague outbreak in 1630 in the tiny town of Monte Lupo, reveals strong conflicts between residents and officials, centered in particular on resistance to official efforts to limit public gatherings.

In Seville, on the other hand, officials met the challenges of plague with temporary health boards created from the existing pool of municipal officials. The men charged with public health duties were therefore much more cognizant of the need to balance a broader array of community concerns with the more specific ones posed by epidemics. These city councilmen were conscious of underlying economic and social issues and were also likely to see a benefit to balancing the various needs of the community as a whole with those of the individuals within it.

One of the most striking aspects of the records from the health commissions in Seville is the benevolent tone of those reporting. Given the strong emotions that plague often provoked, we might expect officials to sound wary, weary, or exasperated by their duties. Instead, there are many striking moments of humanity in their reports. Diego de Toledo, for example, reported from the town of Constantina that "all [who are sick] are poor folk who know little besides hunger and poverty and bad luck has given them this illness."[27] Although members of the health commission, as well as many doctors, often referred to the plague as affecting poor populations most often, there is no blame or stigmatization. Instead, like Toledo, most speak of their lack of proper sustenance or of factors beyond their control, such as the weather. In the same letter, Toledo also recounted the very moving scene of having watched a young girl released from the hospital in Constantina for having no plague symptoms; she left with her sister, shouting joyfully. The incident held no larger importance other than as part of his description of what the town's mood was, but shows a moment he felt worth recording.[28] A short time later, another commissioner, Juan de Perea Durán, reporting on the number of patients admitted to the hospital in the town of La Puebla de los Infantes, also mentioned the death of "a very good nurse whose loss will be deeply felt by the sick."[29] We see most clearly in these occasional comments the humanity of these officials. They did not coldly enforce plague regulations on a population they held in low esteem, but rather worked among a population they felt an obligation to serve properly.

A final important difference between many previous plague studies and that presented here lies in the types of documents available. What gives rise to the documentary evidence that historians rely on are most often conflicts or crises, and plague epidemics tended to provoke both kinds of response. The most common documents related to plague are official ones: regulations on gate closures or guards, decrees of pestilence or quarantine of neighboring towns, orders to create contagion hospitals and convalescent homes. These official statements were often numerous (especially as they began to be printed in the seventeenth century), and therefore are readily found in many archival collections. Many studies of plague, as well as other studies that treat plague epidemics in passing, rely on these official records. Yet these statutes were strict, and when taken at face value paint a picture that is much bleaker than the reality of how they were utilized or enforced. Instead, it is important to read a bit deeper to better understand how these decrees actually affected populations.

This study relies on extensive records from two plague epidemics at the end of the sixteenth century that affected not only Seville, but also the region of Andalucía more generally. These epidemic records are housed in the municipal archive of Seville, the Archivo Municipal de Sevilla (AMS), along with all other records from the city council. The council kept copious notes from epidemics, piling together letters, petitions, reports, and legislative debates into "plague notebooks" (*cuadernos de la peste*). Thanks to a nineteenth-century archivist with an interest in the history of medicine, Seville's municipal archive retains major portions of two of these notebooks, from 1582 and 1600.[30] The earlier epidemic was more localized, affecting parts of Andalucía including Seville, Córdoba, Granada, and the coastal cities including Cádiz and Sanlúcar de Barrameda. Other municipal records show an epidemic beginning in 1580, identified by some chroniclers as *catarro* (catarrh), which waned a bit then resurged by late 1581, increasingly identified as plague by early the next year.[31] The later epidemic of 1599–1600, known as the Atlantic plague, was much more widespread across not only western and central regions of Spain, but also France, England, and the Low Countries.[32] Both epidemics generated a strong official response of monitoring, investigating, and reporting, but both document sets remain clearly incomplete. Both sets begin abruptly when commissioners from Seville were already at work investigating rumors of plague in towns under suspicion, and both sets end while plague was still circulating in both the city and territory; there is no closure for either epidemic. Nonetheless, these are invaluable sources, each set containing over three hundred folios that offer a window onto the range of issues the city councilmen confronted during epidemics. In particular, the voices of residents who experienced both plague and official plague legislation are found throughout both sets of documents.[33] Thus, this study is able to address not only official attempts at control, but also the response of citizens. What is most apparent from these records is constant negotiation between the two.

A second type of plague documentation (conflict) is exemplified by Giulia Calvi in her eloquent study of plague in seventeenth-century Florence. Calvi used the criminal records from the Public Health Magistry in Florence during the epidemic of 1630 to uncover individual experiences, revealing the unexpected effects restrictions on movement could have on ordinary healthy residents. Such residents could and did find themselves facing criminal charges for movements and actions that in other times would have been considered routine and harmless.[34] But where Calvi's documents were created by accusation and prosecution, the documents utilized in this study were created by petition and accommodation, which of course leads to clearly different perceptions and interpretations. Yet the very existence of criminal prosecutions under the aegis of the health board in Florence, which are not found in Seville, points us once again back to the issue of ad hoc versus standing health boards.

Seville as a Case Study

Seville, an important and expanding center of administration, trade, and shipping with the Americas in the sixteenth century, provides a wonderful case study for examining the effects of early modern epidemics on the development of public health. Distant from the immediate environs of the court in Madrid, city leaders were free to enact health regulations or policies as they saw fit, with little direct interference from the crown. Yet there was a balance to be maintained in this respect as well, for the crown used the city's port as its main center to manage the New World traffic, establishing the Casa de la Contratación there in 1503. Therefore the crown maintained an intense interest in monitoring events in the city as it likewise monitored the progress of various fleets sent in and out. The volume of correspondence maintained between the officials of the Casa and the crown, particularly during the reign of Philip II (1556–98), provides additional insight into the functioning of the city during times of plague epidemics.

Seville, like all Spanish cities and towns, had clear routines of governance and public health, which were well established by the sixteenth century. As a center of trade, the city struggled continuously with health threats, and civic leaders were forced to frequently juggle the interests of public health with the interests of maintaining the city's economic and political position. There was simply no way to shut the city off completely from many outside contacts, so officials had no choice but to find compromise among these competing interests. Even King Philip II gave little leeway to fears of plague, refusing to allow his agents at the Casa to remove themselves from the city when they requested to move further south down the river during an epidemic.[35] Among the most important factors influencing civic leaders in their efforts to balance these sometimes competing interests was a variable medical understanding of both the causes of and the best treatment for plague.

Equally important to the city's position as an economic center was its position as an intellectual one. The Casa de la Contratación functioned not only as an administrative body, but also as a central institution for collecting scientific knowledge.[36] Much of that knowledge centered on navigation and cartography, but as Spaniards spent time in the Americas the Casa also became the center of intellectual networks within the city. Among the earliest commodities of the New World that gained interest within Spain were plants used medicinally. Seville had several collectors of these exotic plants and their lore, including two whose publications earned them international reputations for their knowledge, Nicolás Monardes and Simón de Tovar.[37] Additionally, a number of other prominent medical men including Juan Fragoso, Bartolomé Hidalgo de Agüero, and Francisco Sánchez de Oropesa lived and worked there. As practitioners in the city, they treated the residents who were sick and consulted with the city council on matters of public health. As intellectuals, each also published well-known treatises on a variety of medical topics. They also exemplify the larger debates carried on by physicians and surgeons across Europe, as they did not agree fully on the symptoms of pestilence, how best to treat it, or how to prevent its spread. These differences in opinions and experiences also went a long way toward encouraging city councilmen to balance, as best they could, competing interests, opinions, and advice.

The history of epidemics, and especially that of plague, is replete with negative images. Plague narratives most often focus on strikingly pessimistic reactions: of suspicion, neglect, exclusion, and self-preservation. So indeed the response of Seville's city council to news or rumor of plague appears at first glance to be one of fear and suspicion. Seemingly its first action was to shut down several of the city's gates in order to limit access to the city, and to post guards at the remaining ones to prohibit entry to certain people or goods. But a close reading of the records reveals an alternate picture. For although plague remained a feared disease, one finds in the actions of the city council members, specifically those acting as health commissioners, careful investigation, the weighing of evidence, and considered decision making. In all of the reports written by commissioners, none has a tone of blame or disinterest or fear.

Certainly there was still fear and exclusion at both the individual and municipal level. Had no one feared plague, the restrictions on travel and access to the city would not have been imposed. Life was disrupted for everyone by both the fears caused by plague and by regulations imposed by the city council. This is not the whole story, however, and it is important to expand this rather one-dimensional image to more accurately reflect people's attitudes and experiences.

The work of the health commissioners in Seville was vital for helping to maintain some order during epidemics. Whether or not their actions had a medical benefit, their presence in investigating and collecting information reassured residents that authorities were working to protect them. Yet the very measures created to protect residents held their own dangers. The strict enforcement of travel bans and quarantines disrupted trade and communication, endangering the healthy with loss of work, lack of food, or familial separation.[38] These problems were persistent and pushed officials to develop a system that could balance competing interests and concerns.

What emerges from the records in Seville is a view of early modern epidemics that revises our perceptions not only of developments in public health, but also of early modern city governance. Here is clear evidence of a system of administration, and by extension a system of public health, that depended on cooperative efforts by both residents and city officials. City officials, for the most part, upheld the obligations of their job, listening to reports, complaints, and petitions from residents and then investigating before making decisions. Residents, for the most part, recognized the authority of the city council, making the effort to appear before the council to petition for changes or exceptions rather than simply ignoring regulations or taking matters into their own hands. The system wasn't perfect, and there surely would have been breakdowns or occasional corruption. But the overwhelming evidence from two different epidemics is of tremendous effort by both sides to keep the system, and therefore the city, running. Above all, the records from Seville reinforce the well-known, but all-too-often overlooked, idea that one cannot take historical regulations at face value: how authorities wrote laws or regulations was often quite different from how they enforced them. While regulations closing down the city or quarantining an outlying town may seem drastic on the face, closer examination reveals efforts at compromise.

The era known as "early modern" gained that name by being at once both familiar and strangely distant. Times of crisis, including epidemics, offer historians an additional window onto this past, often allowing us unexpected views of both the continuities and differences with our own era.

Chapter One

Early Modern Seville

Balancing Growth and Governance

An Expanding City

The sixteenth century was a golden age not only for Spain as a country, but more particularly for the city of Seville.[1] Spain rose to great power in this century, and Seville played a crucial role in that expansion. As Spain expanded her presence in the Americas, establishing colonies and exploiting resources, an increasing bureaucracy was necessary to oversee it all. In 1503 the crown established the Casa de la Contratación to help manage the emerging shipping and trade with the Americas, as well as to train the ships' pilots who navigated the route and to maintain useful up-to-date scientific and navigational information for this enterprise. The decision to locate this board in Seville, making it the only port through which all ships and their passengers had to depart and return, assured the city's preeminence in Spain and fame throughout Europe. Prior to 1560, Spanish monarchs held no permanent seat of governance, preferring to rotate their court throughout the realm. The mobility of the royal court dated to the marriage of Fernando and Isabel in 1474, which established a joint rule over their respective realms of Aragon and Castile, but did not formally meld the two into one. Instead, the Catholic monarchs treated each territory separately and therefore shifted their court periodically around their realms to oversee governance and ensure their control.[2] It was their great-grandson, Philip II, who chose the small town of Madrid, centrally located but without any previous history of importance that would compete with his vision of power, as a permanent center of government. The growth of Madrid from 1560 on did not diminish the importance of Seville, which continued to expand its leading position in financial, intellectual, and mercantile matters. Though the crown would eventually be forced to relocate the Casa de la Contratación to the coastal city of Cádiz in 1717 as a result of silt in the Guadalquivir River, Seville's reputation as a flourishing city of marvels was by then firmly established.

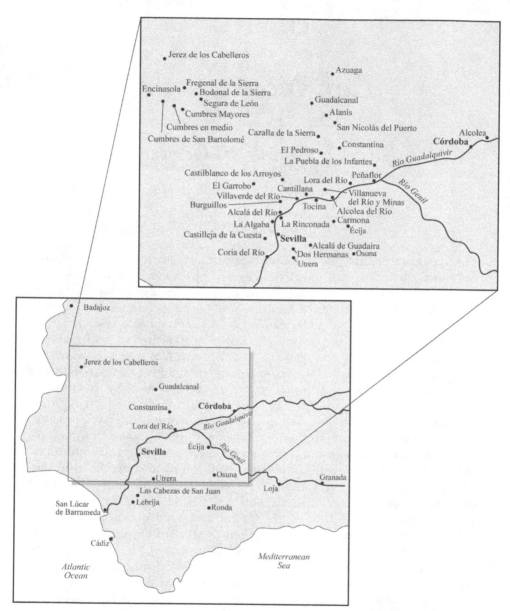

Figure 1.1. Seville and surrounding towns. Map by the Northern Illinois University Cartography Laboratory.

The creation of the Casa and its monopoly meant demographic and economic expansion for the city through most of the sixteenth century. By the end of the century, Seville had grown to become Spain's largest city and the fourth-largest in Europe. Like many early modern cities, there is no clear population data for Seville, so population estimates for the city range between 90,000 and 150,000.[3] This tremendous growth was countered only at the turn of the century, as Seville, along with the rest of Spain, suffered a high mortality rate during the severe plague epidemic of 1598–1600.[4] Seville's position as a trade center made it all the more imperative that the city not succumb to fear or overreact to epidemics, but that it continue to allow as much trade and movement as possible. Throughout the sixteenth century, as the city continued to grow, the city's governing council continued to meet the challenges of not only plague but also other public health issues, much as they had for nearly three centuries.[5]

The city's administrative system had been established in the thirteenth century after Christian forces conquered the city from its Muslim rulers. By then, the city had long been an important commercial center, with roots extending back to the Phoenicians. It was the Guadalquivir River, flowing southwest over fifty miles to empty into the Atlantic, that provided Seville with its vital port. The river was a lifeline and communication route, playing a crucial role in the city from its very beginning. The first Phoenician settlers to southern Spain arrived via the river, led by a sailor and adventurer named Melkart. He set up a commercial warehouse in the area, giving the new colony an economic basis. A legend of the city's founding attributes this feat to the ancient god Hercules. José María de Mena, historian of the city and collector of its legends, argues that in reality Melkart was the person behind the legendary god. Deified after his death, Melkart became known as Hercules and was then absorbed into the Greek and, later, Roman pantheons. Thus it is Hercules who remains the heroic founder of the city.[6]

Through centuries of changes and conquests, the city remained well-situated between land and sea and continued to flourish. Falling under Roman rule, the city retained some prominence within the peninsula. Julius Caesar (d. 44 BC) is said to have kept a residence there, and in later centuries the nearby town of Italica produced two notable Roman emperors, Trajan (r. 98–117) and Hadrian (r. 117–38). The reign of Diocletian (r. 284–305), and the notorious persecutions of Christians carried out in his name, produced Seville's first Christian martyrs, the sisters Justa and Rufina, still popular today as the city's patron saints. As the old Roman Empire fell to the Germanic tribes who overran her borders, Seville, like all of Spain, eventually came under Visigothic control.

Conquered by Muslims along with most of the Iberian peninsula in the eighth century, the city rose to prominence several centuries later under the Abbadid family, *taifa* rulers in the eleventh century. It was the Muslims who built the sturdy walls that encircled and protected the city, pieces of which still stand today. Famous for its olive oil as well as for its manufacturing of musical instruments and ceramic tiles, Seville had easy access to both the large and important Muslim city of Córdoba to the northeast and to the sea to the southwest.[7] The city retained its renown for these products even after being conquered in 1248 by Christian forces led by Fernando III of Castile. The old medieval city with its narrow, winding streets, thick protective walls, colonnades, and palaces, was simply divided into twenty-four *collaciones* (districts or parishes), and land grants were given to those who had participated in the campaign.[8] The city changed little in the subsequent centuries, so that by the sixteenth century it still retained much of its medieval character.

The heart of the old Moorish city became the spiritual and economic center of the new Christian city. The elaborately decorated *Alcázar*, originally built as a fortified residence for Muslim rulers, was turned into a royal residence for Christian monarchs. The mosque that had stood nearby was razed, however, and in its place arose the famous Cathedral of Seville. Built over the course of a century, from 1402 to 1519, the cathedral served as a testament to the city's wealth and piety. The largest medieval cathedral, it remains the third largest cathedral in Europe behind Sts. Peter and Paul in Rome and St. Paul in London. All that remains of the old mosque is the courtyard filled with orange trees (*Patio de los naranjas*), an elaborate entrance wall, and the old prayer tower. The latter was transformed into the bell tower of the cathedral, known as *La Giralda*, still an iconic landmark in the city today.

While the city's port continued to be marked by a Muslim building, the *Torre del Oro*, in the sixteenth century a series of new buildings reflected changing times and the crown's increased economic interest in the city. The creation of the Casa de la Contratación to oversee trade with the Americas prompted a building boom, as the administrative apparatus needed physical spaces to carry out their new duties. The purpose of making one port control all trade with the Americas was, of course, so that the crown could not only control what was shipped out, but also monitor what was coming in. Most important of these imports was the gold and silver brought from American mines, which was quickly taken to the newly created mint (*casa de moneda*) for processing. In addition, the crown needed new spaces for the exchange (*lonja*), and an expanded customshouse (*aduana*), where an important tax, the *almojarifazgo*, was levied on all imported goods. All of this royal interest contributed a great deal to the economic boom of the city itself, providing jobs and helping to expand the infrastructure. These royal offices employed a large number of workers—the customs house alone had nearly 260 employees—used to oversee the collection of import and export duties, the reception and minting of metals from the New World, and all of the administrative paperwork associated with managing the fleets and running the Casa de la Contratación.[9] The population growth, both inside the city and in the nearby towns, prompted a need for easier access to the city, to which the city council responded by expanding the existing city gates and creating new smaller entrances known as *postigos*.[10]

Municipal Government

Despite the crown's role in fostering Seville's development, it remained in many ways a city like any other in Spain, governed largely by local residents who made up the city council. But the economic expansion prompted by the overseas trade also meant that the city itself expanded rapidly. Alongside new buildings for the administration of the Indies trade came new administrative buildings for the municipality. The city government centered around the Plaza de San Francisco, which housed both a new appeals court and the new *Ayuntamiento* (City Hall) designed by architect Diego de Riaña. Here the business of the city was conducted by its governing body, the *Cabildo*, or city council. The city and council were both under the leadership of the *Asistente*, a royally appointed nobleman serving as governor of the city and surrounding towns. The Spanish crown had begun appointing such officials, more often known as *corregidores*, in cities throughout its domain in the fourteenth century, as means of gaining a stronger royal voice in local affairs. These appointments became formalized and used with increased effectiveness under the reign of Isabel I (r. 1474–1504).[11] In Seville, the crown began appointing such officials at the turn of the fifteenth century. These nobles served varying terms, generally of only two or three years each, though some served as many as five or six.[12] The *Asistente* then appointed two assistants, *lugartenientes*, who could stand in during council meetings or on other official business as needed.[13] Presiding at council meetings were the appellate judges, the *Alcaldes mayores*. In the event of their absence, the meetings were run by the *Alguacil mayor*, another royally appointed officer, charged with public safety. The *Alguacil* saw to the proper execution of the judicial system, including supervising the night watch and overseeing management of the jail, which was also located at the Plaza de San Francisco. The judicial system was further intertwined with municipal administration, as the judges for civil (*Alcaldes ordinarios*) and criminal (*Alcaldes de la justicia*) cases were both appointed by the council.[14]

The heart of the city's government lay in the members of the *Cabildo*, made up of *Veinticuatros* and *Jurados*. Originally granted by royal appointment, the position of *Veinticuatro* had become venal and heritable by the sixteenth century, passed along for generations in the same noble families. The name of the office came from their original number, appointed to correspond with the twenty-four parishes of the city. The actual number of officials varied greatly over time, however, never returning as low as the original twenty-four. According to one estimate, by the sixteenth century there were as many as eighty-three *Veinticuatros*, who made up an oligarchy of aristocratic interests.[15] Still, efforts were made to ensure that those who held this position took their job seriously. The city's statutes required *Veinticuatros* to live at least four months of each year in the city, and to attend all city council meetings or pay a fine.[16]

The *Jurados* were parish representatives. Initially two officials elected annually from each parish, they were meant to represent the interests of residents. Abuses crept in here, also, and the positions became lifelong as early as the fourteenth century. Their numbers likewise grew over time, so that by the middle of the sixteenth century they numbered as many as fifty-six.[17] The *Jurados* were required to be members of the lesser nobility (*hidalgos*) as well as residents of the parishes (*collaciones*) they represented.[18] Their job was to handle all city business that affected their respective districts. This included keeping track of households for tax purposes, overseeing the guarding of the city's gates (and the collection of taxes and duties owed there), reporting any unusual occurrences to the city council, and, of course, bringing the concerns of the citizens they represented before the council.[19]

The councilmen were at times also asked to serve on a committee known as the *Fieles ejecutores*. This board was composed of seven men: two *Veinticuatros*, two *Jurados*, two citizens not otherwise employed by the city, and one assistant to the governor, who were collectively charged with maintaining the public order. Their main responsibilities included supervising the public market to ensure fair weights and measures, and overseeing the collection of municipal incomes (*rentas*).[20]

These municipal offices were not simply entitlements or honors, however, and officials were held accountable by both the people of the city and the king. In 1581, when Philip II received a letter complaining that various members of Seville's municipal council had neglected their duties during a recent epidemic, the king demanded an explanation from these officials. The unnamed petitioner specifically addressed the recent actions of both royal officials, the *Asistente* and the *Alguacil mayor*. The *Asistente* was defended as having good intentions ("he has been careful and wishes to do much"), but problems were blamed on his subordinates, who failed to carry out instructions or necessary measures. The *Alguacil mayor* and his deputy were chastised for being absentee, allowing thieves easy opportunities to break into houses. The complaint went on to criticize the city councilmen (both *Veinticuatros* and *Jurados*) for neglecting many of their public health duties, citing filthy streets and lack of sufficient controls to contain the epidemic, such as mandatory burning of clothing and bedding of those who had been sick, and the closing of any houses where deaths had occurred.[21] In response, the king's secretary copied out the text of the letter to send back to the city council, along with the king's demand for an explanation or response. The councilmen did not take these accusations lightly and worked to carefully craft a collective response defending their recent actions and decisions.[22] They retained their positions and no sanctions were imposed, but this likely served as strong reminder that city offices came with serious responsibilities, and those who served in them could be held accountable.[23]

The city council routinely met three times a week, on Mondays, Wednesdays, and Fridays, to handle administrative business. If there was outstanding business to be handled after Friday morning's session, a second afternoon session would be scheduled so that each week would start with new business.[24] In addition to dealing with routine city business, the council heard requests and complaints from residents and visitors, carefully transcribing each into their records. As detailed in chapter 3, these petitions from individuals cover a wide variety of local problems, interests, and issues, and show how individuals who otherwise had little power in the city could gain access to the very highest levels of power. They are a remarkable demonstration of the accessibility of local government in Spain, even in a vast and growing metropolis like Seville.

The power of the city reached far beyond the river and walls that encircled it. In addition to being felt all the way across the Atlantic to the New World colonies, the city's authority was also felt for a large distance into the surrounding countryside. Like all large cities of Spain, Seville controlled an extensive tierra, rural territory dotted with smaller towns and villages. In the sixteenth century, Seville's tierra was generally divided into four sections, the *Campiña de Utrera* to the south of the city, the *Partido del Aljarafe y Ribera* to the west and immediate north, the *Sierra de Constantina* to the northeast, and the *Sierra de Aroche* to the northwest. All together, these regions held nearly seventy towns and villages.[25] According to the city's ordinances, petitions from residents of these surrounding towns and villages were to be heard first, as these citizens would have traveled distances to be heard, while city residents would be less inconvenienced in having to return another day if necessary.[26]

The tierra provided a necessary support system for the city, which depended on the countryside to produce the raw materials and foodstuffs to support a large urban population. Seville's city council had jurisdiction over these towns and villages, though it did not usually intervene directly in their daily affairs. Most often, these smaller settlements maintained their own governance, electing their officials from local citizens, their appointments simply approved by Seville. In some cases, the council intervened more directly, most often by appointing criminal case judges (*Alcaldes de la justicia*) to serve in the larger or more important towns, and occasionally even naming a councilman to inspect or audit a local town council. As shown in subsequent chapters, the council was often likely to intervene in response to epidemics or rumors of epidemics in these outlying towns. At these times, the city councilmen of Seville would take administrative matters into their own hands, sending out their own members with a full range of power to investigate possible outbreaks and to legislate any public health measures.[27] Such efforts were often deemed necessary because of the close ties between city and countryside and the frequent exchange of people and goods that were feared to help spread disease.

The city and tierra formed a tightly interdependent social and economic system in which all municipalities played an important role. The city provided the largest markets to buy and sell all manner of foodstuffs, raw materials, and manufactured goods, and also provided economic opportunities for rural residents willing to work in manual or domestic labor. The towns, meanwhile, depended not only on the city for markets, but on each other as well. The areas of the tierra produced different goods, such as wine in the *Sierra de Constantina*, and wheat in the *Campiña de Utrera*. Intraregional trade provided important links between the various areas, with the city sitting at the heart. Along with overland trade routes, the Guadalquivir River helped tie the region together.

The city's location on the river presented both advantages and problems. The river provided Seville with its secure port, inland far enough for protection of valuable shipments, easily guarded and defensible. It also provided easy connection to the area around it, useful in regional trade as well as long-distance trade. The river and its port also carried continuous traffic not only in goods but also in a constant stream of people and disease. Records of epidemics compiled in the nineteenth century from earlier documents show Seville almost continuously suffering a variety of outbreaks.[28] In addition, a port city is naturally home to large numbers of sailors, transients often notorious not only for their poor manners but also as carriers of disease onshore from their cramped and crowded onboard quarters. Much of the city was spared interaction with the sailors, who preferred quarters closest to the river, many in the neighborhood of Triana. Originating from the days when Muslims controlled the city, Triana lay across the river from the rest of the city and was incorporated as an official parish of the city in 1280, soon thereafter becoming a commercial center.[29] It not only had easy access to the sea trade, but also contained factories producing commodities such as soap and gunpowder as well as painted ceramics and the colorful decorative tiles known as *azulejos*, for which it is still famous today.[30] Triana was linked to the rest of the city by a floating wooden bridge, augmented by private boats used to ferry people back and forth. These individual ferry boats became even more necessary in the face of disasters, as the wooden bridge was susceptible to problems including burning or washing away in floods.[31]

Floods were one of the river's greatest dangers, and presented a frequent problem for the city. At times, the city became so flooded by rains that residents in the low lying neighborhoods needed boats to get around, while those on higher ground were forced to go out on horseback.[32] The city walls, built by Muslims in the days when the city needed fortification and protection from outside attacks, were maintained in part to help block the overflowing river from the city.[33] Reports vary on how many significant floods Seville experienced in the sixteenth century, but it is clear that the city council spent much time and effort working on ways to contain and control the river.[34] This was just one of many ongoing health threats in the city, and councilmen worked diligently to maintain public health in other ways.

Public Health

City councilmen supervised not only the business and trade of the city, but also the health and well-being of all its citizens. The constant ebb and flow of goods and people throughout the city meant Seville faced a large number of ever-present public health issues, from regulation of clean water and food to the provision of medical care for the incarcerated. Behind the glamour of New World riches and the allure of adventure that the city held for many, Seville was also a place whose residents had deep roots there. For them, the city was simply home or market. Though in some cases they had increased opportunities to sell goods and supplies to travelers, their own worlds remained within the city walls. These residents continued their daily lives and relied on the city council to govern and protect them. As part of that, residents had come to expect regulated markets that offered unspoiled and reasonably priced food, some efforts to control the accumulation of filth in the streets, and medical care for the neediest poor.

Public health in the early modern era was reactive rather than proactive, a continuation of ideas and practices inherited from the ancient world. Early modern Europe had continued to accept and develop the humoral concept of health and disease, attributed to Empedocles of Agrigentum in the fifth century BC, codified by the followers of the Greek physician Hippocrates of Cos in the same era, and established as medical canon by the Roman physician Galen in the second century AD. This theory placed greatest emphasis on the regulation of what were termed the six "nonnaturals" to regulate health: air, sleep and waking, food and drink, rest and exercise, excretion and retention, and emotions.[35] As a result, the earliest public health ideals aimed at preventing disease by ensuring, as much as possible, unspoiled air, water, and food.

In Seville, as in all early modern cities, much of what the city council did for public health on a regular basis may be generally categorized into sanitation and management of provisions. The supply of some medical care, particularly for the indigent or incarcerated, was also an important aspect of public health and will be discussed in more detail later. Like all other municipal bodies, the city council of Seville constantly addressed the issues of how to keep streets clean, paved, and passable, and how to ensure provision of sufficient supplies of clean and healthy water and food for the citizens. Urban living provided a variety of challenges to maintaining both good order and good health, and it was to the city council that citizens with concerns about the cleanliness of the city would turn.

> The clergy of the church of San Andrés say that our church has a cemetery in which we bury each year . . . bodies from the parish and the nearby hospital of Amor de Dios and that there are more than 100,000 Christians now buried there[.] In the middle of this cemetery is a large cross, which is a source of great veneration . . . [but] we have often seen dogs removing parts of these same corpses and chewing on them and the residents who live nearby have no respect and throw their trash into it at night[36]

The desecration of cemetaries by dogs was not a common problem, but the accumulation of trash certainly was. The problem of smells arising from trash dumps both inside the city and outside its walls was a constant one. The above petition, which goes on to request that the cemetery be closed to the public, is a good example of the concerns about foul odors resulting from both bodies not buried deeply enough (and hence accessible to dogs) and additional trash thrown in to the open spaces of the cemetery. City council debates in October 1580 centered on both these concerns, as councilmen agreed to order several cemeteries to either rebury bodies or at least to dig new graves deeper, and for quicklime to be spread at the worst of them, including San Andrés.[37]

The council engaged in a seemingly endless battle to keep the city clean. Lacking modern sanitation systems, people discarded trash wherever they found convenient, often in the open spaces of *plazas* or in cemeteries. Like most other early modern cities, Seville suffered garbage-lined streets and clogged gutters, the result of indiscriminate dumping of garbage and waste. The problem was compounded to an extent by the constantly shifting and growing population in the city. Trash heaps, such as that known as the *monte de malbaratillo*, located rather prominently on the main walkway along the river, had accumulated from generations of careless disposal.[38] The outskirts of the city were even worse, as the council maintained little control over dumping there.

Accounts of Seville in the sixteenth century often emphasize this continual battle, with an implication of the futility of city ordinances or official efforts.[39] While this is true, it should also be recognized that councilmen did not give up. Rather than simply continuing to reissue the same regulations and punishments, they tried different approaches to the problem. Some of these changes had little effect in the long run, but they demonstrate the ongoing commitment of city officials to clean up the city. An early city

ordinance imposing a fine of twelve *maravedís* on anyone caught litterir̄
was severe, though largely unenforceable. Through this statute, councilmer̄
hoped to gain popular assistance in enforcing the ban on littering, for if no
guilty person could be found, then the twelve residents living closest to the
trash were to be fined one *maravedí* each. Inspectors hired to maintain watch
and impose the fines proved less than effective, as residents often found it
easy to simply bribe them.[40] By 1640 the situation had gotten out of hand,
and the *Asistente* took matters into his own hands. He sent an inefficient
inspector to jail for his failures, and ordered the city council members to be
held responsible for their districts. Under this system, both *Veinticuatros* and
Jurados alike had responsibility for naming citizens in the different districts
to carry out the clean-up efforts. The residents of each district collectively
paid the costs for these efforts. The trash and refuse collected was taken outside the city walls to specified sites in the countryside.[41] Unfortunately, this
did not solve the problem either, but other attempts abounded, and at least
one successful effort by the city councilmen resulted in the removal of trash
piles and the eventual conversion of a standing lagoon at the north end of
the city into the Alameda de Hércules, a tree-lined park.[42]

The city council also faced problems with street maintenance and frequently received complaints from citizens and petitions for repairs. Paving
of the city's streets did not occur regularly until the late fifteenth century,
when the city received royal permission to impose a tax on meat sales in
order to finance it. Even then, most paving consisted of laying rubble or
unmortared bricks, which led to the need for frequent repairs, some of
which were not simple tasks. One such repair in the late fifteenth century
entailed the removal of 307 cartloads of dirt and manure and the introduction of 489 cartloads of rubble to replace them.[43] By 1525 or so, nearly one-
third of the city's main streets had been paved, and those most important
thoroughfares, meaning those that received carriage traffic, were paved in
bricks mortared with sand or a mixture of sand and lime.[44] Throughout the
sixteenth century, again because of the expansion of population and new
buildings, many streets were reconfigured or expanded. Originally, the city's
regulations called for repairs to be paid for by the citizens "responsible" for
that stretch of road, meaning those whose houses were situated on it.[45] By
the end of the sixteenth century, this rule had been disregarded entirely,
and the city turned again to naming an annual subcommittee of councilmen to oversee the work of cleaning and paving the streets.[46]

While the problems of city maintenance occupied much of the council's
time, of even greater concern was ensuring sufficient supplies of clean water.
The Muslim residents of the medieval city had built public baths, fountains,
spouts, and cisterns, all of them requiring a steady source of fresh water from
outside the city.[47] Once in Christian hands, the city continued its love of water,
distributed throughout the city for both public and private use. Christian

...sidents no longer bathed as frequently as their Muslim predecessors, and ...ne city did not maintain the public baths, but fresh water was still recognized as essential to good health, and the city worked to ensure its continual flow. The city received water not only from the river itself, but also by canals that brought clean water in from the countryside. The most important source of water for the city was a spring at Alcalá de Guadaira, which was brought into the city by the *caños de Carmona*. These carried the water underground in lead pipes for several kilometers, then rose above ground to form an aqueduct at the city gate named for the town it faced, Carmona. These water systems required constant maintenance, and the city council hired two *cañeros* who worked continually to keep the waters flowing into the city as needed.[48]

The other essential for good health was fresh food, particularly grain. In times of scarcity, the city relied on supplies stored in the *alhóndiga*, the public granary, to supplement or replace poor harvests. When these reserves ran low, it became necessary to import grain from distant parts. Grain transported overland was generally believed to be healthier than that imported by sea. There are frequent references to the poor quality and dangers inherent in grain brought in via sea routes, known as *trigo del mar*.[49] Other foodstuffs could also be suspect, and the city council carefully guarded against the importation of wine and olive oil coming in from the countryside in times of plague, inspecting any goods and sometimes requiring they be examined by a doctor to ensure their quality.

Like other local officials in the early modern era, Seville's councilmen contracted a number of medical practitioners on both a continuing and sporadic basis. These included a wide range of practitioners: physicians, surgeons, nurses, and a variety of specialists such as bonesetters and cataract removers. The expanding economy and population in Seville meant a greater demand for health care. While most health care in the sixteenth century remained private, an increasing number of poor residents found themselves unable to afford treatment. For those already dependent on the municipal government because of poverty or incarceration, this meant a need for doctors and surgeons willing to treat them.

Seville was the crossroads between the Old and New Worlds, the first stop on the way to a new start. It drew a constant stream of visitors and travelers, most of whom passed through, but some of whom decided, for one reason or another, to remain. For the city council, this presented both problems and benefits. On the one hand, it meant an influx of people seeking opportunities, not all of whom would be able to find them. On the other hand, the city also attracted capable and trained medical specialists looking for opportunities. Some sought a quick fortune, others sought careers, but all sought opportunity of some sort.

In 1604, Mathias de Ayala, a professional bonesetter employed by the city council of Seville to treat the poor, petitioned the council for a raise in his yearly salary. Ayala was, by this time, a longtime resident of the city. He had arrived some twelve years earlier as a visitor, passing through on his way to the Americas to make his living practicing medicine. Instead, he found himself employed in Seville and stayed to make his home there. Ayala recounted all this in his salary petition, going on to point out that although he was originally hired to work alongside another doctor, Hernando González de Contreras, he had in fact been working alone for several years. Dr. Contreras had left his original municipal position for another one, becoming the doctor at the royal jail located in the city. Ayala carefully reminded the council of the opportunities and salaries from other places that he had forsaken to remain in Seville, and he asked for an additional 50 ducats per year, bringing his annual income to 200 ducats.[50]

Ayala's position in the city reflects not only municipal concern with health, but also the strong royal interest maintained in the city. Only two years prior to his arrival, the position of bonesetter had been established by royal mandate. In response to what were perceived to be an excessive number of deaths resulting from untreated broken bones (often suffered in falling from mules), the crown had ordered the city to hire an *algebrista* or bonesetter to care for the poor who injured themselves, paying his salary from the municipal income (*propios y rentas*).[51] It was this position that Ayala fell into and carried out diligently for many years.

Along with specialists such as Ayala the bonesetter, the city government employed a range of full-time medical practitioners to care for the poor and incarcerated. Several of the full-time medical employees of the city council worked at the royal jail located in the city. The city paid salaries not only to a physician, but also a surgeon, barber (phlebotomist), pharmacist, and nurses. When one of these positions opened up, the city council would accept letters from prospective applicants and vote by secret ballot on the candidates. Once named to a position on the municipal payroll, it became incumbent on the employee to send a written application to the city council for the pay due to him for the previous year, two years, or in some cases of procrastination, four or five years. Upon receipt of this application, the city council would take it under advisement, assign a council member to check that the applicant had indeed fulfilled his duties for the time asserted, and order payment only when satisfied that the job requirements had been fulfilled. In most cases, salaries were paid without much fuss, though occasionally questions were raised.

When disputes arose, the employee accused of dereliction had the opportunity to defend himself. When Pedro García Arroyal, a surgeon at the jail, was initially denied his requested pay because of charges that he had not properly attended to his job duties, he prepared a written rebuttal. He argued that he did indeed carry out his assigned duties, visiting the jail daily to attend to sick prisoners and asserted that those few days on which

he did not visit the jail were times when there simply were no inmates needing his treatment. In addition, García Arroyal presented the city council
with testimonies from the jail supervisor, Jácome Fernández, and two of the
doormen, Francisco de Morales and Pedro González. All three testified that
García Arroyal had faithfully attended the sick of the jail, visiting even two or
three times a day when necessary.[52]

Disputes such as this were the exception rather than the rule, however,
and once appointed to one of these positions, the same person could continue in that capacity for as long as he wished to remain there, though the
council could, of course, easily remove anyone they deemed unfit to continue practicing. It is not unusual to see the same doctor, barber, or nurse
employed for fifteen, twenty, or even thirty years by the city. In many cases,
municipal appointments were not granted to young practitioners, but rather
to older, more experienced ones. Thus, it often occurred that the same person held a position until his death.

In 1623, Francisco Chaves took over as barber for the jail, charged with
bleeding patients as needed, both as health remedy and preventive measure.
He held this position for many years, receiving his salary in lump sums every
three or four years. Ten years later, he was still on the job and took on an
assistant to help with the duties at his pharmacy, a young man named Pedro
Gómez. After twenty-one years serving the city as barber, Chaves died. Upon
his death, his widow applied to the city and received his back salary due.
She also appealed to the council to appoint her late husband's assistant,
Pedro Gómez, to the newly opened position as barber. After due consideration, including a consultation with the physician to the jail, the city council approved Gómez, with only one dissenting vote. Four years later, Gómez
applied for the position of jail surgeon, a job separate from that of barber.
He was one of four applicants, and was not awarded it. The surgeon who was
awarded the job died two years later, and Gómez was then successful in his
second application. The arrangement seems to have suited both the council
and Dr. Gómez, as he served both positions for the next twenty-eight years,
applying every few years for the respective salaries to each position. The surgeon's position carried far more prestige and a better salary than that of
barber, as Gómez earned 20,250 maravedís per year as surgeon, and a mere
8,000 maravedís per year as barber.[53]

City positions were open to women as well as men. Agustina de la Cruz
was a beata who worked at the women's prison as a nurse. She began working
for the city in 1635, at a yearly salary of 12,000 maravedís.[54] She continued
to work in the jail for over thirteen years, receiving an annual salary. After
her death, her widowed sister, Doña Catalina de Quizada, applied to the
city council for the back pay owed her deceased sister and was granted it. In
addition, she also applied to take her sister's place at the jail. She was eventually granted the position, but her petitioning process reveals the slowness of

some council actions. They appointed a councilman to look into her request in August of 1647, but did not officially grant her the position for another eight months.[55]

Not all practitioners were so fortunate as to find gainful employment in Seville. Fernando de Meneses, a trained physician, moved to Seville from the city of Salamanca. He came in search of work, moving his family with him. Although he was able to demonstrate his credentials as a reader of philosophy, astrology, and medicine for six years at the University of Salamanca, he could not find employment in Seville and eventually petitioned the city council for charitable assistance.[56] Another unsuccessful case, that of Diego de Tovar, shows the range of backgrounds of those who appeared before the city council. Tovar was a Portuguese soldier, traveling through Seville in 1569 on his way to fight in Granada where the *Moriscos* were in revolt. Upon his arrival in Seville, however, he found parts of the city suffering an outbreak of disease. Out of great compassion, he distributed his own formula of medicinal water among the sufferers at no charge to them. He then alerted the city council to this great generosity by way of his petition for recompense from them. Arguing that he had provided a great service to the public, Tovar pointed out the council's obligation to repay his kindness as well as their duty to the citizens not to let him be lured to another city. The council's response was not enthusiastic, though they did duly appoint a small commission to investigate his claims. As no payment was made, and nothing seems to have been heard from him thereafter, it is likely that he found opportunities elsewhere.[57]

By the sixteenth century, the city of Seville was a flourishing and dominant urban center. With urban growth came urban problems, and the city council increasingly expanded the scope of their efforts to keep the city relatively clean and to provide access to clean water and food. Residents were not always compliant to regulations and councilmen faced an ongoing battle, one that required persistence, patience, and sometimes ingenuity. As a regional center, Seville dominated the tierra around it, providing both opportunity and supervision to the many small towns within. The routines of city government, of commerce and trade, of markets and exchange, and of health care, were all well established. The greatest threat to these routines came from pestilential epidemics, which could decimate populations and endanger trade routes. But even for plague, Seville's councilmen worked out a system of response that allowed for flexibility and, in the long run, stability and prosperity. This system of response to epidemics was predicated on the early modern understanding of health and disease, a complex set of knowledge vastly different from the modern one.

Chapter Two

Perceptions of Plague

Balancing Disease Concepts

Early Modern Plague

Coping with plague in the early modern era required a multifaceted balancing act by both officials and residents. Although not all the balances discussed in this and subsequent chapters were performed consciously or with foresight, in the end they nonetheless achieved their unacknowledged goal: to protect individual health while also protecting the health and functioning of the community. To do so, officials found themselves struggling to balance a variety of needs.

The next chapter will explore the actions of the officials as they sought to keep the city running as smoothly as possible. To better understand those actions, however, it is necessary too understand the context in which they were undertaken. Therefore, this chapter examines the variety of beliefs about plague—what caused it, how it spread, who was at risk to contract or spread the disease, and how best to treat the sick—that informed the decisions of city officials. Much like today, public health decisions were rarely simple and nearly always involved balancing health interests against other social and economic needs. Medical officials rarely diagnosed an epidemic as exclusively plague. Instead, they often saw multiple sicknesses, which they termed plague (*mal de peste*), typhus (*tabardete*), or simply a general contagion (*mal contagioso*). The signs that physicians looked for to diagnose pestilence, including the bubo (*landre*) and carbuncle (*apostema*), could be identified as "pestilence" or "contagion," but the terms themselves were not unique to plague. An *apostema* to early modern Spanish doctors could simply be an abscess that would drain and heal, a *landre* could be any tumor or swelling. Thus, even diagnosis involved its own form of balancing symptoms, signs, and prognosis.

Early modern conceptions of disease embraced a multiplicity of causes, as exemplified by the most famous description of the plague, that by Giovanni Boccaccio in his introduction to *The Decameron*. Set in Florence in 1348, the

work is fictional and may be seen as more emotive than factual in the descrip‑
tions it offers. Yet it also provides insight into the ways that Europeans, from
their earliest experiences with plague, sought the causes of disease in a wide
range of factors:

> Some say that it descended upon the human race through the influence of the
> heavenly bodies, others that it was a punishment signifying God's righteous
> anger at our iniquitous way of life. But whatever its cause, it had originated
> some years earlier in the East, where it had claimed countless lives before it
> unhappily spread westward, growing in strength as it swept relentlessly on
> from one place to the next.
>
> In the face of its onrush, all the wisdom and ingenuity of man were unavail‑
> ing. Large quantities of refuse were cleared out of the city by officials spe‑
> cially appointed for the purpose, all sick persons were forbidden entry, and
> numerous instructions were issued for safeguarding the people's health, but
> all to no avail. Nor were the countless petitions humbly directed to God by the
> pious, whether by means of formal processions or in any other guise, any less
> ineffectual.[1]

Although written in the mid-fourteenth century, Boccaccio's descriptions
of beliefs and actions were still accurate in many ways over two centuries
later. This passage neatly encapsulates the various aspects of medieval and
early modern medical understanding: the moral effects of God's wrath, the
environmental effects of a dangerous planetary alignment, the miasmatic
effects of filth and refuse in the streets, the threat of contagion from allow‑
ing the sick to enter the city. In addition, despite the best efforts of residents
to prevent what they could, Boccaccio points out the disease "swept relent‑
lessly on," as if an entity unto itself.

Nearly three centuries later, an account of an epidemic in 1649 in Seville
shows a similarly multifaceted understanding of plague. Francisco de Ruesta
was pilot major for the Casa de Contratación from 1633 to his death in
1673. His account of this epidemic discusses first the distant cause of plan‑
ets, citing the influence of "malevolent" planets and eclipses observed in
Valencia and Murcia in 1646 and 1647. This created the pestilence, which
he explains then spread to the port cities of Andalucía (Santa María, Cádiz,
and Sanlúcar) by means of contagion (*por contagion*). Seville was hit hardest
by the epidemic, which arrived in infected clothing at the port, once again
"augmented by the influence of malevolent planets," principally Saturn and
Mars. He goes on to recount how the air of the city was further corrupted
by excessive rains that April, which swelled the Guadalquivir River, causing
"stomach upsets, much nausea and vomiting" (*grandes alteraciones de estomago,
y muchas nauçeas, y vomitos*) which in turn led to "attacks of buboes, tumors,
carbuncles (both simple and complicated), and typhus, which seized them
so violently that they died in two days, one and a half, a quarter of a day,

~~nstantly."[2] A variety of causes, both environmental and man-made (trade goods, travel), all leading to a plethora of woeful symptoms.

These descriptions of diseases, symptoms, and their causes as emerging from multiple sources, some controllable by man and others not, reflect a view of disease that has long been lost to modern thinkers. This multiplicity of sources has often posed problems for historians attempting to understand responses to plague in the early modern era, for belief in multiple causes of disease creates a seemingly chaotic response pattern. A clearer understanding of how early modern thinkers perceived the causes (and potential causes) of disease can make those response patterns somewhat more intelligible.

Plague stood out as a diagnosis for early modern thinkers as the ailment that killed more people more rapidly than any other, but physicians responded to the visible symptoms as they would to any other set of symptoms, fitting them into the existing intellectual framework of humoral theory. This framework, resting on assumptions of balance, was a flexible one that incorporated ancient ideas of both individual response to environment and contagion. An ancient concept, "contagion" was another flexible term that was used as often metaphorically to describe the spread of heresy, for example, as it was literally to describe the spread of disease.[3] Early modern thinkers faced the challenge of further refining this fluid concept of contagion to fit both their existing conceptual framework of disease and their experiences with plague.[4]

Developed first in ancient Greece as a Hippocratic movement and later associated with the second-century Roman physician Galen, the humoral theory offered a comprehensive explanation for the workings of the human body and its interactions with the larger natural world. The four basic humors (blood, phlegm, black bile, and yellow bile) that made up the body, existing in unique ratios within each person, gave shape to both physical and emotional temperaments. The humoral ratio, subject to daily and seasonal fluctuations, had to be carefully monitored and adjusted in order to ensure good health; excessive imbalance resulted in disease. Just as these humors could be characterized by their qualities—degrees of hot, cold, wet, and dry—so also could the resultant symptoms of imbalance. Treatment, then, relied on rebalancing either through addition of what was lacking or depletion of the excess. In this understanding, diseases were not discreet ailments brought about by distinct causative agents as we understand them. Rather, a simple imbalance could shift from benign to dangerous, turning what seemed a routine ailment into one later deemed "pestilential." These beliefs were, of course, a result of long experience. In the age before antibiotics, simple scrapes could indeed lead to severe infections, simple coughs to pneumonia, and any fever was cause for concern.

While individual symptoms or ailments could easily be explained through diet or lifestyle, widespread or epidemic illness presented additional problems of explanation. The association of weather or climate with health is an ancient one, likewise traceable to the Hippocratic corpus of the fifth century BC. This belief took two related forms. First, it was accepted that the climate of a particular area affected the temperament and overall health of the population living there. For doctors (and residents) in Seville, treatises such as Juan de Aviñón's *Sevillana medicina* and Juan de Carvajal's *Suma de los nueve mil y treinta y cuatro peligros a que se sujetan los naturales y vecinos de Sevilla* (Summary of the nine thousand and thirty-four dangers to which citizens and residents of Seville are subject) offered an examination of the "air" of the city, the diseases to which residents commonly fell prey, and the regimen of treatment best suited to them.[5]

In addition to this overall influence, however, came a more immediate effect of changing weather that could negatively influence individuals who were previously healthy. Such links figure prominently in reports from Seville's health commissioners. Juan de Perea Durán, for example, writing from the town of La Puebla de los Infantes in 1582, asserted in his report that "with these cloudy days, three or four more women have fallen ill."[6] Similarly, a doctor in the town of Constantina reported "on the 23rd [of January], the air of this town being tempestuous and for this reason, very pernicious . . . resulted in four illnesses. On the 24th the weather cleared and so there was only one further illness."[7] These and other similar references throughout the epidemic records reflect one of the contingencies that officials continually juggled, the ties between atmosphere and pestilence. Plague treatises throughout the early modern era emphasize the primary role of "tempestuous" air in causing disease. Alonso de Freilas, for example, in his 1605 study on plague, lists simply three causes of plague: the will of God, the planets and their influence, and the air we breathe.[8]

Air, in particular the corrupted or poisoned air known as a miasma, was the primary and most crucial explanation for the spread of many diseases, including plague. According to miasmatic theory, air became polluted or poisoned by any number of factors, including a dangerous alignment of planets (first cited by the Paris medical faculty as the cause of pestilence in 1348 and routinely pointed to by authorities in later epidemics), unusual natural phenomena such as earthquakes, and local factors, such as accumulated garbage that created noxious (and therefore unhealthy) smells.[9] Foul odor was a sure sign of corruption of the air, so all urban smells increasingly came under scrutiny and suspicion, including the work of odiferous professions such as tanners and fish mongers as well as the everyday accumulations of household refuse, chamber pots, and miscellaneous street filth. These smells were considered the immediate or local cause, and one that local officials often focused on, because it offered the most immediate possibility of remedial action. Men could do nothing about planetary alignment, but they could certainly clean streets.

At the same time, both medical and lay officials had long embraced the idea that plague was also contagious, that it spread via contact or proximity with the infected. As defined by the medieval writer Isidore of Seville (c. 530–636), "Plague, *pestilential*, is a contagion which, when it takes hold of one person, quickly spreads to many."[10] Observations of the patterns of infection gave increasing credence to these beliefs as families or households suffered illness and deaths in quick succession.

While contagion itself was not a new theory, plague prompted new considerations of how disease could spread so quickly from one person to another. Specific understandings of how plague could be contagious were not easily or quickly worked out. Galen had proposed a concept of contagion via small "seeds" of disease that could pass from one person to another. But later thinkers used this idea only to explain small-scale local transmissions of diseases such as colds, pneumonia, scabies, or even leprosy.[11] Isidore of Seville's discussion of plague asserts that, "It arises from corrupt air, *corrupto aëre*, and by penetrating into the viscera settles there." He goes on to say that "it is called 'contagion,' *contagium*, from 'touch,' *contingere*, for whomsoever it touches, it infects."[12] This helps explain the dual concept of miasma and contagion, but does little to explain the patterns of illness observed from the fourteenth century on. Later writers continued to wrestle with these issues of transmission. An anonymous treatise from Montpellier in 1349, for example, asserted that plague was caused by poisoned vapors, which from inside the body may emanate through the eyes. Then, "if a healthy person sees this visible vapor, he is stamped with the pestilential sickness." The author goes on to suggest "from this we may conclude that we should above all take precautions against the gaze and breath of people in the throes of illness."[13] Throughout the ensuing centuries, medical writers continued to offer new or refined versions of contagion theory, even as municipal authorities enacted public health regulations predicated on an undefined means by which plague spread via contact or proximity.[14]

Further complicating the issue, as Ann Carmichael has demonstrated, different authorities could invoke different or even conflicting meanings of contagion.[15] These varying definitions and beliefs can certainly make modern studies more difficult, but they should also be seen as simply adding to the mosaic by which early modern people understood all disease, including plague. For early modern thinkers, ideas of contagion could be held distinct from those of miasma at times, but were most often closely entwined with both miasma and humoral imbalance. While the specifics of how disease could pass from one person to another remained under speculation for centuries, what mattered most was the response this idea prompted: separation of the sick and healthy. While the original quarantine, first implemented in the Venetian trading colony of Ragusa (Dubrovnik today), was a means of ensuring that ships did not unwittingly bring plague into the harbor, the idea of using quarantine to separate from the general population not just those at risk of developing sickness but also those already sick, became increasingly popular after Boccaccio's time. Over the next few centuries, as communities continued to deal with pestilential epidemics, another potential cause of disease gained greater prominence. Through the fifteenth century and into the sixteenth, intellectuals increasingly associated the outbreak of disease, particularly plague, with poverty.

Ties between plague and poverty did not emerge in the earliest fourteenth-century plague epidemics, but developed in the fifteenth century. Historians have long examined these links, describing the response to plague as increasingly based on social rather than medical issues. Examining plague in Florence, Carmichael argues for a social shift in attitudes toward the poor in direct relation to the spread of plague epidemics. Florentines became "certain that poorer people, especially migrants and beggars, were carriers of the disease. There was a deepening conviction that plague and poverty were linked threats to the security of the state."[16] Likewise, Brian Pullen, examining sixteenth- and seventeenth-century Italy, argues for a "kind of dualism" in which the poor were both "subjects of pity and objects of fear," considered "the incubators and spreaders of disease."[17] Paul Slack argues that by the seventeenth century, local English officials began to recognize patterns of infection that centered in poor areas. Plague became "a problem potentially greater and more personally threatening than the problems of poverty, vagrancy and suburban disorder; but it was a problem linked with those other social diseases and similar in kind to them."[18]

The connection between plague and poverty existed as well in Spain, but a close reading of the documents in Seville reveals a more complex and more benign interplay of factors. The poor (and vagrants) were always a concern, but the connection most often drawn by Seville's officials was one of poverty leading to poor food, which left the poor more vulnerable to disease. As a result, while sixteenth-century Spaniards believed the poor were prone to *developing* disease, they saw little wider threat of the poor to *spread* disease to the healthy. By seeing (consciously or not) the health threat as one of diet rather than miasma or general environment, health commissioners enabled a delicate balance to continue. Crises could be managed with greater ease as city officials charged with investigating rumors of illness both within the city and in the smaller towns of the tierra held little fear in visiting these sick poor, confident that they were in no danger themselves. By remaining unconcerned for themselves and diligently carrying out their various duties of investigation, city officials managed epidemics effectively, thereby keeping residents calm and reassured.

During the epidemic of 1582, Diego de Toledo, a councilman investigating rumors of plague, reported to the health commission from the town of Constantina, stating that "all here are very poor and know nothing except hunger and poverty and bad luck has given them these problems."[19] Half a century later, a chronicler of the city described the conditions that led to plague spreading into the city from surrounding areas in 1649. The author recounts the common concern over Triana, the busy neighborhood of the city that sprawled across the opposite bank of the Guadalquivir River, apart from the rest of the old city. While officials worked to protect the rest of the city from plague by closing gates and posting guards to interrogate travelers, they could do little more than mount sporadic patrols around the perimeter of Triana, a much less effective means of monitoring movements. According to the author, the 1649 outbreak spread from the countryside first into Triana, then quickly moved from there to neighborhoods "up against the walls of the city, areas inhabited by the poor and beggars."[20] He then adds that it would be "impossible to avoid introducing the disease into the city because there are many who live in these neighborhoods, whose houses and tenements are home to the official poor and beggars who must have access to the city in order to feed themselves, and although the contagion is not carried on their persons, it certainly would come in their clothing."[21]

These quotes offer distinct views of the causes of plague, but both effectively illustrate that although early modern Spaniards associated disease with poverty, they did not blame the poor for their plight. Poor relief was an obligation that could not be ignored, and the chronicle's description is particularly striking for its acknowledgment of this obligation, even to those who may bring disease with them. Here again is a strong contrast to what is more often documented, the rejection of or blame of the poor as spreaders of disease. This alternate perspective of the poor is a reflection, perhaps, of the conservation of different kinds of documents rather than a reflection of different character. Attitudes are never ubiquitous, but we can only access them by interpreting the pieces of evidence left behind. This makes it all more imperative to bring these alternate views to light in order to better grasp the full range of attitudes or beliefs.

In part, this different attitude of toleration for the poor may be attributed to shifting ideas about poverty in the sixteenth century. Reviving older medieval ideas of classifying the poor into categories of those who could not work versus those who would not, municipal leaders across Europe began to reevaluate traditional systems of poor relief.[22] Beginning about 1520, officials in many cities sought to organize (or reorganize) official channels of charity, replacing traditional forms of private charity with public ones.[23] These reform movements sought to classify the poor, acknowledging the responsibility of those in power to those who were "truly" needy. In movements to separate the able (and therefore "lazy") poor from those genuinely unable to support themselves (the "deserving" poor, such as the lame or widows), both royal and municipal officials sought not only to act as good Christian leaders, but also to reduce the larger threats to public order that widespread unregulated poverty was believed to encourage. One of the best-known treatises arguing for this classification was that of Juan Luis Vives, whose 1526 treatise, *De subventione pauperum* (On assistance to the poor), was written for city officials in Bruges where the Spanish expatriate lived. But there were numerous other works discussing the problems of poverty and recommending charitable remedies. Within Spain, influential treatises from Miquel Giginta (c. 1543–88) and Cristóbal Pérez de Herrera (1558– 1620) toward the end of the century resulted in the creation of numerous new hospitals or houses for the poor, which aimed to provide work for the able and support for others. Though the reforms advocated by many were not long-lasting, facing financial difficulties in the seventeenth century, the impetus for new poor relief programs based on registration and classification remained strong through the second half of the sixteenth century.[24]

Seville participated in this movement, undertaking reforms at the end of the sixteenth century at the request of the crown. In 1597, city officials rounded up nearly two thousand poor residents to be inspected and licensed for begging if they were found truly needy. Yet this was apparently not an effort to limit the number of beggars in the city, for by one account the city had prepared nearly double this number of begging licenses.[25] This process of categorizing individuals offered legitimacy to those deemed worthy, enabling Christian charity to continue without concern for "freeloaders." In part, this system of licensing the poor may have helped contribute to an ongoing acceptance of the "official" poor as part of the city, whose need for assistance outweighed any health threat they could pose.

The strong association of hunger and plague recurs frequently in the records from Seville. In February 1582 when officials from the town of Cazalla de la Sierra sent a series of reports to the officials in Seville, they all stressed the effects of hunger rather than contagious disease. Diego Sanchez Cornado, a clergyman, asserted that "if any persons have died in recent days they were poor and died of pure hunger and lack of foodstuffs."[26] Doctor Salvador Esteban agreed that "the people who have died were very poor and miserable," asserting that "it is certain and true that men from outside may enter and do business without fear of contagion and that the principle cause of illness here currently is a lack of food."[27] Reporting from the town of La Puebla de los Infantes, Juan de Perea Durán referred repeatedly to "the lack of bread, which is great."[28]

Similarly, in April 1582, officials in Seville called together a number of the city's medical practitioners to ask their opinions as to whether plague cases existed in the city, and specifically whether the city ought to commandeer houses or other buildings outside the city walls to use as a plague hospital where "pestilential" cases could be isolated from contact with others.[29] Fourteen medical practitioners, including doctors, doctor-surgeons (*medico y cirujano*), and apothecaries (*boticarios*), testified they were currently treating several patients. Their diagnoses varied, however, some asserting having seen cases of plague, while others insisted the illnesses were "usual for this time of year" but not specifically "pestilential." Yet all agreed that it was the poor who were sick. In the words of Doctor Diego de Tamayo, "the people who now suffer this illness are poor and do not have the means for treatment, and those that I have treated and visited are very poor."[30] Doctor Benito Carrero suggested the city should "order these poor be treated by two or three doctors," and nearly all the others likewise refer at some point to the poverty of those who were ill. The men who seemed to support a plague hospital did so on the grounds that the poor could be better cared for there, and specifically because they would receive better food there. Their testimonies reflect no sense of panic or even concern that an outbreak of plague was imminent; rather, their focus was on providing better sustenance, which, in turn, would reduce the incidence of disease. There is no sense in these testimonies that such measures should be undertaken to protect the wealthier or better-fed population, who presumably are not at risk in such circumstances. In response, the health commission followed Carrero's suggestion, ordering a dozen local doctors to visit and treat the sick poor in the various parishes of the city, and to report back any signs of plague.[31]

In all these reports, the tone is one of obligation to the poor as needing assistance rather than one of fear or blame of the poor for harboring disease. Seen in this light, the willingness of Seville's officials to first impose restrictions and then negotiate their selective enforcement (as discussed in detail in the next chapter) can be interpreted not as a reflection of negligence or ignorance, but rather as a reflection of the often shifting concepts of how plague erupted and how or why it spread among populations. Certainly, when tied to issues of nutrition, plague became a more manageable and less threatening disease.

Yet even this link between plague and nutrition or starvation remained under some debate. Certainly all the major outbreaks of plague in Andalucía during the sixteenth and seventeenth centuries were associated with times of famine. Scarcity of grain, the staple of diet for all classes, resulted from a variety of factors including drought, swarms of locusts, and the requisitioning of Seville's supplies by the crown to supply royal fleets.[32] Yet while officials often blamed simple starvation for leading to disease, the real problem cited by many others was that times of scarcity resulted in the need to import grain, often shipped by sea. And it was this grain, known as *trigo del mar*, that many blamed for causing disease.[33] The practice of shipping grain was common, and it was certainly still much easier and cheaper to move large quantities by sea than overland.[34] So it seems largely during epidemics that officials, doctors, and clerics alike proclaimed the dangers of *trigo del mar*. According to city councilmen, such wheat held a "bad odor" and caused "the said contagious diseases as well as many others."[35] Juan de Flores, a clergyman in the city, petitioned the city council for action on two aspects of danger for residents in Seville. The first was their consumption of *pan del mar*, which he described as bread either made from bad flour mixed with good, or in worse cases, used full strength. The second danger was that of filth in the streets, particularly the unusually large number of dead cats and dogs, which caused a foul odor to fill the city.[36] This concern with *trigo del mar*, shared by many in society, did not disappear quickly. As late as 1784, Don Cristobal Jacinto Nieto de Piña, a member of the Royal Medical Society of Seville, published a thirty-page study entitled "Discussion of Wheat Flour, Its Conservation and Method to Distinguish Good from Bad," in which he likewise refers to the dangers of transporting wheat by sea, still then an easy and common form of transport.[37] This may not have been an unreasonable concern, as it is now recognized that grains, including wheat, when stored under damp conditions, can grow toxic fungi including ergot. Such molds or fungi would have likely contributed to mortality rates at any time, and may indeed have stronger links to plague mortality rates.[38] Nonetheless, in times of absolute scarcity, officials often had little choice but to import wheat from whatever source they could, simply one more balancing act they faced periodically.

Plague and hunger went hand-in-hand in the early modern era, one seemingly provoking the other in a vicious cycle of escalation. In Andalucía, news (or even rumor) of an outbreak of plague, regardless of whether attributed to tainted air, water, clothing, or grain, generally provoked a quick response of municipal quarantine. Surrounding towns and villages quickly moved to assess the threat to themselves, issuing orders when necessary that travelers and goods coming from infected areas be denied entry. The cities of the area, including Seville, Córdoba, Carmona, and Granada directed these quarantines, but they extended throughout the countryside down to smaller villages. As a result of such quarantines, not only were residents prevented from traveling outward to other cities, but often all trade coming into the infected town stopped as well. In the words of a surgeon in Cazalla de la Sierra, "the greater problem is hunger, because the supplies we usually depend upon are not delivered."[39] This exacerbated the problem, as the poor, either starving or eating low-quality food, could thereby increase the plague rate, creating a vicious cycle. Yet many officials seem to have recognized this, often advocating either for municipal quarantines to be lifted (allowing the resumption of normal trade) or for the provision of better food to the poor.

The following chapter focuses on such efforts by officials to ameliorate the worst effects of both plague and plague restrictions. But in order to effectively weigh their actions, officials relied not only on their observations and experiences, but also on the medical knowledge of doctors and surgeons around them. These medical experts provided strong opinions and suggestions of guidance for the best approaches to protecting public health. Unfortunately, they presented just as varied a set of beliefs, each informed by both their medical training and their experiences in past epidemics. Thus, the expertise they offered simply reinforced the multiple understandings of plague.

Spanish Medical Authorities

The varied ideas, discussed above, of what caused plague and how it spread reflected similar debates among medical authorities, both those who published treatises (of which there were many) and those who simply practiced in their communities, whose voices can be found in municipal records. The humoral system in which all physicians were trained was based on notions of change and fluidity, which led to varying interpretations of both diagnosis and prognosis. By the sixteenth century, numerous Spanish universities offered courses in medicine for study beyond the bachelor's degree. These included Salamanca, Alcalá de Henares, Valencia, Zaragoza, Seville, and Granada.[40] Study in these medical programs, like those across Europe in this era, centered on studying the theory of ancient authorities including Hippocrates, Galen, and Celsus, as well as more recent texts and glosses from Islamic scholars such as Avicenna.[41] These texts, of course, often presented theories of health and disease in broad terms that left room for interpretation, and how to apply that textual knowledge to actual practice also left room for debate. By the early modern era, then, there were many medical issues under contention including diagnosis, prevention, and treatment of a host of ailments. Plague (*peste*) remained at the forefront of most-feared epidemics and therefore continued to receive frequent treatment in published works. The extensive list of plague treatises produced not only in Spain but also across Europe testifies to the variety of interpretations, opinions, and beliefs regarding the prevention and treatment of plague.[42]

The publication of medical treatises in sixteenth-century Spain centered in the university towns of Salamanca, Alcalá de Henares, and Valencia, the court in Madrid, and the ever-expanding city of Seville. Seville's publishing houses, led by the famous Cromberger family, added a considerable number of texts to an already crowded field.[43] In addition to a handful of texts on plague published in Seville in the early part of the sixteenth century, the plague epidemic of 1599–1600 prompted another eleven authors to publish their views. Many of these authors wrote in Spanish rather than Latin in order to access a wider audience, especially surgeons or other practitioners without knowledge of Latin, trained through apprenticeship rather than in universities. While Spanish surgeons began some studies at universities in Spain or Italy by the end of the century, most continued to be trained as craftsmen rather than intellectuals. Throughout the early modern era, many Spanish medical authorities engaged in a larger ongoing debate over the validity of using the vernacular for medical texts.[44] In the case of plague, however, few dissented with the need for a broad-based sharing of knowledge to understand and combat epidemics. Some, including Luis Mercado, even went so far as to publish editions in both Latin and Castilian.[45]

Plague treatises published in Seville during the sixteenth century continued to put forward a variety of arguments about the causes of and best treatments for pestilential epidemics. While nearly all plague treatises offered a standard set of possible causes, from the alignment of planets to air corrupted by accumulated garbage, others engaged in a series of disputes over the nature of pestilence and the best means to treat it. One such dispute centered on treatments for plague, including purgatives and bleeding. Although many prominent authors, including Juan Carmona, physician to the Inquisition in Llerena, and Luis Mercado, court physician to Philip II and *Protomédico* (head of the crown's medical licensing board), defended these treatments, others disagreed, notably Cristóbal Pérez de Herrera, a royal advisor and physician to the royal navy best known for his work on poor relief, *Discursos del Amparo de los legitimos pobres* (1598). In 1599, Pérez de Herrera published a work on plague questioning several popular treatments, from diet to phlebotomy. Other medical authors in Seville joined this dispute, including Andrés Zamudio de Alfaro and Andrés Valdivia.[46]

Of perhaps greater influence than disputes over bloodletting as treatment were more fundamental questions of what constituted plague and whether plague should be considered contagious. Francisco Sánchez de Oropesa, writing in Seville, argued strongly in his treatise *Tres proposiciones . . . a la ciudad de Sevilla, en que se ponen algunas advertencias para la preservación i cura del mal que anda en la ciudad* (1599) that plague was not contagious. In a new edition and expansion of a previous treatise on plague (*Tratado de peste*, 1569), Sánchez de Oropesa argued in this later edition against the contagious spread of plague based on his observations during an epidemic in 1581. At that time, he asserted, he had seen clothing and bedding from plague patients reused without spreading disease, leading him to believe that plague did not spread through such means.[47] Although strongly supported by another local practitioner, Juan de Saavedra, Sánchez de Oropesa nonetheless faced tremendous opposition from others, including his colleague Zamudio de Alfaro.[48]

Little wonder that civic officials struggled to make sense of epidemics and establish policies when even medical authorities disagreed on causes, spread, and treatment. Many of the authors of these treatises were also active practitioners in the city, consulted by the city council for their diagnoses and prognoses of epidemics. Thus, these disputes were not merely theoretical debates carried out in print; they were the ardently held beliefs of local medical men in the city, whose differences of opinion made the job of city councilmen that much more difficult.

The April 1582 meeting of doctors with city councilmen discussed above included two men who were already published authorities on health matters, Nicolás Monardes and Francisco Sánchez de Oropesa. Two others who testified in April would go on to publish their own treatises at the turn of the century (alongside Sánchez de Oropesa's new edition), Fernando de Valdés and Bartolomé Hidalgo de Agüero.[49] These were men whose opinions had a direct impact on the debates over policy and yet represent only a fraction of the voices that clamored different viewpoints in the sixteenth and seventeenth centuries.

In testifying for the health commission in 1582, each practitioner stated how many patients he was then treating and what he had diagnosed. Opinions varied widely among them as to the presence of "pestilence" within the city, some affirming having seen suspicious cases, others insisting that the fevers they treated were merely typhus (*tabardete*) or other common seasonal illnesses. In one somewhat confusing testimony, Doctor Martín de Busto declared that he had "visited and treated many people, and although it is true that I saw a number of cases of pestilential illnesses (*enfermedades pestilenciales*) and dangerous symptoms such as *gomitas* common with typhus (*tabardete*), which are signs of a venomous humor, but none of the said patients had any buboes, none of them died, and this illness is of an ordinary sort for this weather."[50] He went on to affirm his belief that these patients were not a threat to spread disease. The weather, according to this doctor, could apparently cause illness that while pestilential was also benign. His colleague Diego de Tamayo, on the other hand, affirmed having treated five cases of what he called plague (*mal de peste*), of whom three had died.[51] Bartolomé Hidalgo de Agüero, a surgeon at the Hospital del Cardenal, who had by 1582 a well-respected reputation in the city, and who would insure his posthumous reputation with the later publication of an impressive surgical treatise, concurred with Tamayo.[52] He, too, had treated four cases that he identified as plague (*mal de peste*) in recent days, three of whom had died. He went on to affirm that alongside plague, however, numerous residents also suffered other ailments he identified as *modorras*, *tabardete*, and *tercianas*. For Hidalgo de Agüero, these were common ailments and even the deaths from *peste* were not enough to warrant setting up a quarantine hospital, for fear of the scandal it would cause both within the city and in surrounding areas.[53]

Other doctors offered a similar variety of opinions. Most asserted a range of illnesses present in the city, some affirming and others denying pestilence. Most agreed that publicly building or establishing an isolation hospital would create a scandal and escalate fears both within the city and in surrounding areas. Officials, both lay and medical, generally resisted acknowledging a plague outbreak until absolutely necessary, in the interest of protecting residents from being ostracized by other cities and maintaining trade levels unimpeded. Yet several doctors also admitted that isolated treatment centers would be beneficial, if the city could quietly commandeer houses outside city walls without provoking public attention.

The next month, the commission assembled another group of medical personnel for further testimonies on the health status of the city, this time calling together those physicians and apothecaries the commission had ordered to visit and treat the sick poor through the various neighborhoods of the city.[54] This second meeting included some of the same men, including physicians Benito Carrero and Nicolás Monardes and apothecaries Rodrigo del Castillo and Juan del Valle. Also attending were nine other physicians and four other apothecaries. Here again, the men did not agree on whether the city faced an epidemic of plague. Monardes staunchly denied the presence of plague in the city, insisting that too few had died to merit calling this illness plague.[55] Others, including Drs. Carrero and Gaytan, stated that there was not an outbreak of plague in the city, although there were some "pestilential illnesses."[56] Still others insisted that many residents remained sick and this illness should be identified as plague.

Such disagreements in diagnosis played out on the individual level as well, making the task of the health commission occasionally more complex. On March 22, 1582, after hearing of a sick child in the parish of San Roman, the health commission sent the constable Alonso Rodríguez to accompany the surgeon Jorge Suárez in checking on her illness. Suarez found young Isabel, who he described as a child of eight or nine, to be suffering a malignant fever and symptoms of plague. Rodríguez dutifully contacted a local pharmacist for the necessary treatments and the health commission authorized payment to Isabel's mother of 6 *reales* for her to buy necessary food for the child. The following day, however, a second surgeon argued to the health commission that he had examined Isabel and found her only suffering a mild fever with no signs of plague. In response, the commission did not further concern themselves with her case, simply filing the records of this investigation in with others.[57]

With such inability to form a consensus, it is little wonder that city councilmen relied as much on their own judgment as that of doctors. When Gonzalo Martín, a wine merchant in the city, fell ill after returning from a visit to Constantina in late January 1582, for example, he came under the health commission's watchful eye. Constantina had been declared infected only ten days previously, which made Martín's illness of some concern. The city's governor, the Count of Villar, sent Diego de la Peña to visit Martín to confirm whether he had been visiting Constantina, and to verify his illness.[58] Peña visited Martín the same day and also spoke with his doctor, Bartolomé Hidalgo de Agüero. Questioned about Martín's illness, Hidalgo de Agüero told Peña that his patient had an open sore in his groin and a fever, but no other symptoms of plague. His professional opinion was that Martín did not have plague or any other "dangerous contagion." Peña, however, was concerned by Martín's admission that he had returned sick from Constantina nearly eight days previously, so he ordered Martín and his wife, María Hernández, to remove themselves to a house outside the city walls, and then closed their house in the city.[59] Martín and his wife remained in their new residence outside the city for three weeks before petitioning the commission to be allowed back into their home. Martín asserted that his sore had healed and he showed no other signs of illness. He asked the health commission to again consult Dr. Hidalgo de Agüero, who had continued to treat him during his exile. This time, upon taking Hidalgo de Agüero's testimony confirming Martín's complete health, the commission approved his petition, and allowed him and his wife to return to their house unimpeded.[60]

City officials charged with establishing public health orders faced the challenge of weighing this variety of opinion against what they deemed in the best interests of the community, attempting to negotiate a difficult path between creating unnecessary scandal and letting an impending epidemic get out of hand. In order to successfully accomplish this, it was necessary to ascertain exactly where the sources of infection were, and who did or did not pose a threat for spreading plague. Neither question was an easy one, but officials worked to find the best possible answer to them. The variety of opinions regarding the cause and nature of plague provided officials with room to continually reshape their own attitudes and practices. The plague legislation enacted by these city leaders shows one important part of this continual effort, for it demonstrates a starting point of how officials worked to protect the city.

Responding to Plague

In light of this multiplicity of beliefs regarding the causes of disease, early modern civic officials initiated programs of public health that attempted to address as many of these beliefs as possible. Like their counterparts across Europe, Seville's officials in the sixteenth century utilized a program of response to plague influenced by this varied understanding of disease, but still strongly grounded in the techniques of response developed in earlier centuries.

While no plague outbreak affected all of Europe in the same way the first pandemic of 1348 had, nearly all cities continued to experience local outbreaks that appeared at least once a generation. Seville, for example, experienced at least fourteen significant epidemics recorded by either medical or municipal authorities as pestilential during the sixteenth century, some seemingly lasting two or three years as symptoms (and mortalities) subsided then reemerged seasonally.[61] By the sixteenth century, the ongoing experience of Europeans with the waxing and waning of epidemics enabled them to develop routines of response. As Paul Slack has pointed out, the initial crisis of the Black Death was far too overwhelming for any governing bodies to establish organized response. Instead it was in later years with the continual development of smaller, somewhat less lethal epidemics that governing officials found the time and ability to develop public health programs.[62]

Historians have long pointed to the Italian city-states as forerunners in their creation of what became the standard system of response to plague. The earliest plague outbreak (1348–52), now often referred to as the Black Death, progressed rapidly and visibly across Europe from Mediterranean ports inland. This progression led to the earliest beliefs that people and trade were bringing or carrying disease with them, though the exact mechanisms remained debated, as demonstrated previously. The first response of Italian leaders in the fifteenth century, therefore, emphasized efforts to limit contact between sick and healthy, a regimen that depended first and foremost on maintaining communication networks so that cities could gain early warnings when plague had broken out in other areas.[63] Motivated as much by politics as by public health concerns, leaders of the Italian city-states created boards of health that are often credited as being an important part of the first systematic attempts to monitor and preserve public health.[64] When civic authorities declared an outbreak of plague in an area outside the city, they quickly closed city gates, leaving only one or two open for traffic. Guards posted at those few open gates demanded that travelers present health certificates for both themselves and any merchandise they carried, verifying their town of origin and health. The encircling walls and gates of cities, built in the Middle Ages to thwart invading armies, were now utilized against invisible enemies of disease.

When they found plague inside the city walls, municipal officials isolated the sick (and sometimes their families or households) either within the home or in designated isolation hospitals (*lazaretti*). Officials worked to further break the chain of infection by fumigating houses and burning the clothing and bedding of the infected, regardless of whether they recovered or not.[65]

Such practices, adopted initially as temporary measures in these Italian territories, eventually shifted to become standard across Europe. While some areas outside northern Italy, particularly Aragon, which had long-standing political and cultural ties to Italy, created permanent boards of health, nearly all municipalities adopted the same kinds of measures on a more impermanent, periodic basis.[66]

The *Comisión de la salud*

> In the city of Seville Friday the 20th of April in the year 1582 the city council being gathered according to custom the illustrious gentleman don Fernando de Torres y Portugal count of Villar and governor of this city along with several gentlemen of the council . . . the council orders that a subcommittee of the plague commission shall be formed because for the past several days there have been a number of suspicious illnesses in the area . . . [they are to] give an account to the city on these matters and new commissioners should be named to deal with these matters . . . the same group should work on all that pertains to cleanliness in the city as a matter of greatest importance to the overall health of it.[67]

When plague struck, or even threatened, the city of Seville, the city council utilized a response program that, while ad hoc, was also adaptable and effective in allowing the city to continue to function during epidemics. It centered on the naming of a plague commission composed of city councilmen and headed, like the council itself, by the *Asistente*. These plague commissions were temporary bodies created, revised, and disbanded as needed. The commissions in Seville varied in size, and were subject to change during any given epidemic. The commission referred to in the above quote was twenty-five men, a group explicitly named as a smaller committee than previous ones. In truth, the task of the plague commission was a daunting one—to monitor health in the city and throughout the municipal territory at both the collective and individual levels. To this end, they often met separately from the full council, had their own clerk, and maintained full control over all matters relating to the epidemic, from gathering information to issuing restrictions and payment orders.

The councilmen named to handle issues relating to epidemics became known as *diputados de la peste*, or plague commissioners, who worked with a relatively small group of doctors to investigate, treat, and control plague outbreaks. A handful of these commissioners were mobile; if there were illnesses and deaths in the towns of the tierra, they spent time traveling to the infected towns and villages of the countryside, monitoring health and imposing precautions and restrictions there. The remainder stayed in the city, forming a sort of base of operations that investigated within the city, collected the information filtering in from the city and countryside, evaluated it all as best they could, and issued instructions and restrictions accordingly.

Within the city, commissioners worked continually to gather and evaluate information for two purposes. First, they investigated health risks posed by sick residents in the city, or anyone attempting to enter the city without authorization. Second, they investigated the circumstances surrounding individual petitions before either granting or dismissing them. In this way, the commissioners worked continuously to balance the need for supervision of the community with various other needs of individuals. In doing so, they also became public symbols, observably and diligently monitoring people and goods in the name of public health.

Sixteenth-century Spain was still primarily an oral culture, in which people learned news by public announcement and word of mouth. It is no surprise, then, that the health commissions relied a great deal on rumors and word of mouth for information. News passed not only laterally through neighborhoods or from town to town, but also vertically, so that word of a suspicious illness in a home or inn quickly reached the highest levels, prompting investigation. Although the health commissioners had no formal system of surveillance—no standing health board, no permanent investigators, no paid informers—they don't seem to have needed them. Instead, the commissioners relied on local networks, augmented by medical practitioners to provide diagnoses and medical assistance. Commissioners ordered local physicians, surgeons, barbers, and apothecaries to report any known or suspected cases of plague during epidemics, with, of course, a threat of stiff monetary penalties for failure to do so.[68] Likely, they also relied on reports of suspicious illness from parish officials and fearful citizens.[69] While some of this verbal chain has been obscured by time, what remains visible in the council records is a seemingly omniscient *Asistente* who instigates these various investigations with the formulaic phrase "it has come to my attention." Once this information reached the commission, however, it became documented. Commissioners then acted as detectives, calling witnesses, recording testimony, and in other ways collecting information. They went out into the streets, checking on reports of suspicious illnesses, meeting with doctors, and tracking down visitors to ensure they did not pose a threat of spreading disease. While we have no way of knowing how many things escaped official notice, the commission's records reflect constant attention and effort to monitoring and maintaining the health of the city. Along the way, their records offer a rich and varied source of information on many aspects of daily life in the city.

But beyond mere observation and investigation, the commission also held real power. Headed by the royal governor, it commanded respect both inside and outside of the city. The commission's financial powers included issuing payments to both individuals who assisted the city during epidemics (doctors, pharmacists, and guards, for example) and to towns in financial need. Plague commissioners also held appointive powers, sending doctors and surgeons to work in distant towns of the tierra as needed. They could delegate their powers in the towns of the tierra, appointing a local official as *juez de comisión*, which gave him temporary power to act locally on behalf of the commission.[70] Most important, the commissioners controlled travel and trade within the municipal territory. They issued bans and quarantines, granted exceptions to them, and ultimately decided who was or was not a health threat.

> We agree to notify the guards of all the gates of this city that they shall not allow entry to any persons who come from the towns of Constantina, Cazalla de la Sierra, and La Puebla de los Infantes, nor allow any clothing or textiles of which they have reason to be suspicious that they arrive infected with plague[. We also agree] that Señor Luís de Herrera shall write a letter in the name of the city to Licenciado Perellón, the judge in the town of Constantina, requesting that he work with all care and diligence to cure the illnesses of plague in that town.[71]

Once city officials received sufficient news or rumors of a plague outbreak to warrant the creation of a health commission, their initial task was generally to determine the extent of the threat. This meant delegating commissioners to visit surrounding towns and villages, collect direct information, and alert local leaders of their newly suspect status and the need for residents there to avoid traveling about the countryside.[72] They also began to contact additional towns, particularly those that lay along the travel routes between the city and infected towns, checking for cases of plague and ensuring that officials there were on the alert not to let travelers from infected towns pass through.[73] In addition, they sent commissioners out to continue gathering information on suspected outbreaks of plague in other towns.[74]

Only in 1582 was the issue of religious response broached by the city officials, when commissioners, after consultation with the archbishop, ordered that in all parishes, as well as the cathedral, priests were to say prayers for the preservation of those towns already infected, as well as for the continued health of the city itself.[75] It's unclear why the commissioners in this case decided on such a decree, as prayers were nearly always a part of any response to epidemics, but rarely mandated by the secular government.[76] The breadth and depth of the religious response is reflected in several city chronicles, including that of Diego Ortíz de Zúñiga. He carefully described the various religious processions carried out in the city, including one in June 1582 that included images of the city's patron saints, Justa and Rufina, as well as images of the patron saints of plague, Sebastian and Roque.[77] Other chronicles likewise record formal processions and supplications, reflecting the importance of prayers and processions during epidemics.[78] The vast majority of this religious response, however, was neither organized nor promoted by the city government. Despite giving earliest attention to matters of prayer, the health commission was actually little concerned with a religious response to plague. Aside from this brief mention, the commission never again gave any direct orders relating to spiritual matters or sponsored any religious actions. Instead, it concentrated on more concrete actions for keeping the city as healthy as possible.

In both 1582 and 1600, as the epidemics increased or spread, the commissioners issued a formal set of regulations as they attempted to stem the expansion of the disease through a variety of measures. In 1582, these regulations were recorded as usual by the city council's scribe, but by the later epidemic in 1600, the regulations were printed.[79] While this may seem a minor change, it would have meant an enormous change in the accessibility of these regulations—which gates were open and closed, where patrols were posted, and what documents were necessary to gain entrance to the city. The number of city gates left open (and monitored by officials) varied. In 1582, it was just four: the Puerta de Carmona, Puerta de Arenal, Puerta de Macarena, and the Puerta de Triana, which were open at 5 a.m. and closed at 9 p.m., guarded day and night by members of the city council.[80] Limiting the number of gates one could use to enter the city ensured careful monitoring of who was coming into the city and what goods they brought with them. Guards questioned everyone wanting to enter the city about where they came from and what business they had in the city, and turned away anyone traveling from towns known to be infected. Any market goods they brought with them, including wine, vinegar, textiles, or grain, would likewise be refused entry. Travelers who produced a "health certificate" verifying that they came from a town known to be healthy gained entry. In 1600, efforts to monitor travel were expanded outward as the newly printed regulations stated that the commission would name commissioners to serve at seven local stopping points (inns) outside the city. These commissioners would interrogate all travelers, allowing only those with proper documents showing their most recent place of residence to move on to the city proper.

Having issued orders that aimed to combat plague brought on by God's anger or by wayward travelers, the commission next turned its attention to a final important source of disease, that of the environment. As discussed previously, this was the most common belief of the cause of plague. The solution was first to clean the streets and then to purify the air. The commission in April 1582 thus ordered the purchase of twenty-four carts and twenty-four mules, which were to be used throughout the city to thoroughly clean the streets of all refuse.[81] In the epidemic of 1600, the commission also paid for quantities of rosemary and thyme to be distributed to the various parishes for public burning in order to purify the air.[82]

As an additional measure of caution in the 1582 regulations, the health commission interviewed a number of doctors regarding the cases they had treated within the past fifteen days.[83] As discussed previously, they did so to gauge the threat of plague within the city walls, and to gain expert opinion on the necessity of setting up isolation hospitals for treatment of the infected. The city council only utilized such plague hospitals sporadically, particularly during large-scale epidemics within the city.[84] During the extensive epidemic of 1599–1601, for example, the city ran two plague hospitals and a convalescent home. The commission generally used the Hospital de Cinco Llagas (also known as the Hospital de la Sangre), which recently had been built just outside the northern end of the city (outside the Macarena gate) in 1540, as one isolation hospital. They then commandeered space for an additional hospital and for a convalescent home in Triana. Thus hospitals were accessible but technically outside of the city limits.[85] In other cases, rather than creating and maintaining specific plague hospitals, commissioners simply ordered that residents remove themselves from their homes, dictating only that they move outside the city walls, not to a specific location.[86]

According to the doctors consulted in 1582, the city at that time was facing a combined epidemic of plague (*peste*) and typhus (*tabardete*). Typhus was another common cause of epidemics in the early modern era, first described in Spain in 1489–90 during wars to capture Granada from Muslims. It was far less feared than plague, because it was far less deadly.[87] By modern understanding, typhus is spread by body lice, which would travel easily in clothing or other textiles. While this was certainly not recognized at the time, a diagnosis of either plague or typhus prompted at least one common response—the avoidance of textiles (clothing and bedding) as possible sources of infection. Experience and observation of patterns of infection had shown that such textiles seemed to increase the spread of disease. Thus one of the first measures taken in times of plague was to forbid entry of persons or cloth from infected areas. Similarly, the response to both plague and typhus was to ensure that all clothing and bedding owned or touched by an infected person, regardless of whether or not they survived, be burned. Woolen fabrics were thought to harbor one form of contagion, and fire was believed to be the one sure means of purifying and removing the contagion.

From a modern perspective, this may not have been a bad strategy, as heavy woolen textiles would have easily contained infected fleas and lice. For people in the early modern era, however, burning was a costly and often seemingly unnecessary measure. Families with few resources often sold extra clothes and bedding to dealers who would re-dye them and sell them secondhand. Even some hospitals routinely participated in this market. Throughout the year, for example, administrators at the hospital of Cinco Llagas collected the unclaimed clothing of any who had died there. Once a year they sold this clothing, using the funds they obtained to sponsor masses for the souls of the dead as well as for charity gifts. In those years of plague, however, they suspended such sales, noting in their records the prohibitions on resale of cloth.[88] By ensuring the burning of clothing and bedding of plague victims, the health commission eliminated a small source of income for some needy families, cut into dealers' income, and prevented the poor from obtaining cheap secondhand textiles. Many attempted to circumvent the restrictions against reselling textiles belonging to those who had been sick, and the health commission received frequent complaints about such efforts.[89] It was important, therefore, that the commission at least see to replacing destroyed items for those who recovered from their illness.

This then, was the standard municipal approach to plague epidemics in Seville, used for centuries. It differed little from that implemented by other Spanish cities, or indeed of most other European cities.[90] It was a multifaceted approach to preserving health, but one that relied most heavily on isolation and limiting contact with possible sources of contagion. Yet the legislation itself tells only half of the story. The other half can only be found in the debates, decisions, and actions of the councilmen that both preceded and followed the creation of this legislation. In particular, the councilmen's willingness to continually amend their plague legislation reflects their ongoing efforts at balance.

Chapter Three

Negotiating Public Health

Balancing the Individual and the Community

Negotiating Exceptions

In the town of Castilleja de la Cuesta . . . Diego de Escobar, resident of the city of Seville and visitor in this town, . . . [states that] I have been in this town and the town of Manzanilla . . . more than ten days . . . and currently I am healthy and away from any danger of illness or contagion [I ask that] these witnesses I present be examined [to confirm this].[1]

In late January 1582, Seville's city council sent word across one section of its tierra, the territory to the northeast known as the *Sierra de Constantina*, informing local leaders in the towns there of newly imposed restrictions on travel to the city. Those leaders in turn sent out town criers to announce the new restrictions in the public plazas, and city councilmen in Seville ordered similar announcements be made in the city. At each of the city gates around Seville, authorities notified guards and posted on public bulletin boards the names of towns newly declared suspect of harboring a plague epidemic. The towns of Constantina, La Puebla de Los Infantes, and Cazalla de la Sierra were now under suspicion, their residents and any goods from the area forbidden entry into the city. For many of Seville's residents, the news simply added to the worries of pestilence that seemed to swirl almost permanently through the area. For the previous two years, disease had stalked the residents of Seville and the tierra steadily, often diagnosed as *catarro* (catarrh).[2] While today this would refer to influenza, it is less clear what the sixteenth-century diagnosis meant. In any case, it was not considered pestilential and apparently required no great investment in public health efforts. Yet for many other residents, these new restrictions in 1582 hit home, disrupting their routines of travel and forcing them to find alternatives.

For Diego de Escobar, a wine merchant from Cazalla de la Sierra ready to haul his wine to the city for sale, the new restrictions meant using some creativity to accomplish his goals. Unwilling to simply sit idly until the quarantine on his town might be lifted, Escobar instead used his resources and his knowledge of the politics of public health to gain exemption from the restriction. As a resident of Seville's tierra, Escobar knew that he could gain access to explain his case before the city council, asking for permission to sell his wine within the city despite his town of origin. But to help ensure his success, he astutely worked to provide the city council proof that both he and his goods were healthy and therefore would pose no risk upon entering the city. The quarantined towns were all located in the northeast section of Seville's tierra, while the rest of Seville's territory remained unrestricted. So Escobar hired carters to carry his 334 *arrobales* (approximately 1,423 gallons) of wine to the outskirts of Seville, but did not travel with them.[3] Instead, Escobar traveled directly west to another part of Seville's territory known as the *Aljarife*. There had been no suspicious deaths recorded in the towns there, and Seville's city council had not placed any restrictions on the movement of those residents. After passing a couple of weeks visiting friends, Escobar petitioned a judge in the town of Castilleja de la Cuesta for an official declaration of his health. He made no secret of his town of origin and why he was asking for this document. As part of his petition, Escobar presented the judge with three witnesses who all vouched for the time he had recently spent in town and for his continued good health. The judge granted Escobar his declaration of health, though he was careful to include the details of Escobar's story and his plan to gain entry to Seville by obtaining a health declaration from outside of Cazalla de la Sierra.[4] Armed with his document, Escobar gained permission to enter the city. He waited another two weeks within the city before petitioning the council for permission to bring his wine within city walls. In his second petition to the council, he carefully pointed out that by this time the wine had been sitting for a month and a half outside the city, more than the usual forty-day quarantine required to determine health.[5] In response, the health commission of the city council asked the local doctor Bartolomé Hidalgo de Agüero to inspect the wine. Upon receiving Hidalgo de Agüero's declaration that the wine was fine to bring into the city, the council agreed to Escobar's request, though with the caveat that the wine had to be decanted into vats brought out from the city and transported only on mules likewise from the city.[6]

Diego de Escobar made a rather complex effort to circumvent official plague restrictions, and was able to do so through his knowledge of the system of quarantines and his acquaintances in other towns who allowed him to visit. But in his overall determination not to let restrictive legislation interfere with his business, and in his use of the open channels of communication with Seville's city council, he was far from unique. In fact, just a week after enacting the restrictions of January 1582, the health commission received the first of a steady stream of petitions from individuals seeking special permission or licenses to either enter the city or bring goods into the city despite the restrictive legislation. Over the course of four months, from February through May 1582, the health commission received nearly fifty such petitions from individuals. Perhaps most surprising is that council-men were not only willing to receive and evaluate these requests, but they also granted each one. While we might expect residents to address com-plaints to their local councilmen, the complicity of the health commission in allowing continual exceptions to the very restrictions they had just put into place is striking. Moreover, this process of restriction, petition, and exemption was not unique to the spring of 1582, but was repeated again in 1599–1600 as well as throughout subsequent epidemics of the seventeenth century.[7] Throughout the early modern era, the "closed" gates of the city were remarkably porous.

This pattern of enacting then contravening protective legislation seems oddly contradictory to modern minds and raises a number of questions. In his journal describing the plague outbreak of 1651 in the city of Barcelona, Miquel Parets suggests that a doctor sent to diagnose whether an outbreak was plague may have been bribed into declaring it was not.[8] Could Seville's magistrates have been likewise bribed into continually contravening their own directives? While this pattern could be interpreted as simply a careless approach to public health, a better understanding of their actions lies in a more nuanced understanding of public health in the early modern era. As shown in the previous chapter, diseases were perceived as much more complex in the early modern era than currently and even physicians often didn't agree on diagnosis. At the same time, Seville's city leaders were con-cerned with more than simply avoiding disease, they also needed to protect the overall well-being of the community as a whole. This included protect-ing economic stability and traditional rights of residents. The restrictions passed during plague epidemics were aimed at protecting the community, but could also be detrimental to individuals like Diego de Escobar, who found themselves caught between their own economic needs and the city's legislation. The city council's willingness to allow continual exemptions to its own legislation reflects a recognition of this problem and an attempt to balance the needs of community and individual.

Certainly, people remained fearful of plague, and for many the mere mention of the disease would have been enough to create worry. But for many others, like Diego de Escobar, outbreaks of plague became one more variable for which one had to plan, and perhaps merited some caution but did not stop one's economic and social routines of travel and trade. The vast flood of petitions sent through the city council testify to the resil-ience of the population of Andalucía (though surely they were not unique in this respect) and their determination to continue their lives even with plague circulating. People remained strongly attuned to news or rumors of illnesses that could be plague, and they continued to report to officials suspicious behavior or suspicious illnesses, but they did not stop their daily routines of work, market, or other travels, both within the city and across the countryside, in the meantime. Whereas fourteenth-century chroniclers emphasized social breakdown as a result of the constant flight of people away from infected areas, by the sixteenth century officials were far more concerned with attempting to control the movements of people into infected areas. The records from Seville reveal repeated cases in which travelers and merchants moved without concern across territories where numerous towns had been declared infected with plague. While the officials were concerned that such travelers could spread disease, the travelers themselves appear remarkably unconcerned that they might encounter disease. By the sixteenth century, people had grown sufficiently accustomed to plague that news or rumor of epidemics in and of themselves no longer caused economic and social breakdown.

Yet while early modern responses to epidemics became increasingly routine, rational, and flexible, the image of plague as a destroyer of social and economic systems has remained. Laurence Brockliss and Colin Jones, in their discussion of plague in sixteenth- and seventeenth-century France, assert that "plague . . . was not simply a disease, it was the harbinger of death—even death itself—stimulating fear, dread, and panic." Their summary of plague treatises from this era reflects an even more dire impact: "the plague-stricken town was like a gruesome pastiche of hell, where the visible and olfactory superabundance of rotting human flesh signaled the sundering of normal bonds of sociability. Trade stopped; streets emptied; empty houses were looted; and in a generalized atmosphere of *sauve-qui-peut*, children were abandoned by their parents, aged relatives by their family, masters by their servants."[9] A vivid image, certainly, but one entirely unsuited to sixteenth-century Seville. For while Spaniards recognized their ultimate inability to predict or fully control outbreaks of plague, they nonetheless sought policies of response that specifically prevented such breakdown.

Redefining Public Health

Sandra Cavallo, in her study of charitable systems in early modern Italy, was the first to suggest a modified scheme for assessing public health, suggesting that historians must begin to include the importance of symbolic efforts alongside assessments of medical or material efforts to prevent plague.[10] This reinterpretation alters traditional notions of the "effectiveness" of plague legislation to include its social or psychological impact, a valuable starting point to discovering balance.[11]

Thus, while Seville's health officials seemingly negated the medical effectiveness of their plague restrictions by granting continual exemptions to them, those same exemptions provided an effective means of balancing health concerns with economic, social, and psychological ones. City officials acting as health officers maintained trust from residents in two seemingly contradictory ways. First, they enacted the same sort of restrictive regulations (i.e., travel bans and quarantines) that most authorities, both civic and medical, believed to be the best means to prevent the spread of plague. Such official action offered peace of mind to residents and reassured them that administrators were working to protect them. But by the sixteenth century, experience had shown that while uniformly stopping all travel and banning trade goods might help stop the spread of disease, it also created new crises that could be just as, or even more, detrimental to public health. Thus Seville's regulations, while aimed at the preservation of material health, can also be seen as symbolic, for officials never enforced them completely. Instead, the city health commissioners worked on a nearly case-by-case basis to evaluate when to enforce this legislation and when to allow exceptions. Those who complied with restrictions, using official channels of communication or accepted methods to seek exemption, generally succeeded in obtaining allowances; those who attempted to (or even appeared to) circumvent these accepted methods faced official scrutiny and possible detention in jail.[12] Officials used their presence as investigators to both reassure and warn residents of the seriousness with which they took their public health duties. But it is important to recognize that officials didn't simply arbitrarily decide when to enforce the rules, rather, they created formal channels through which residents could apply for (and often gain) needed exemptions from legislation. Officials did not simply impose restrictions on residents, instead, they worked cooperatively with them to balance the fears of plague with the needs of residents. Their ability to keep peace and order rested on their ability to maintain this delicate balance. The exemptions they granted likewise held both symbolic and material meanings. By allowing residents to voice their concerns and circumvent restrictions, officials not only provided symbolic reassurance that individual residents were not powerless, but also provided concrete ways that residents could avoid suffering unnecessarily from those restrictions.[13]

Along with investigating possible sources of contagion, plague commissioners spent equal or more time investigating the circumstances surrounding petitions. Despite clear orders from the health commission that anyone attempting to enter the city had to carry papers proving their town of origin and their health, most people lacked such papers. Instead, they simply petitioned the commission for permission to enter or to bring in whatever goods they carried with them. One of the most distinctive aspects of Seville's plague response is the frequency with which residents sought and received such exceptions to plague restrictions. One might expect, perhaps, to find such exceptions granted to the wealthy or well-connected residents of the city. In addition, the commission received numerous petitions from merchants asking permission to import wine, grain, timber, textiles, or other goods. Their willingness to grant these petitions is understandable, for granting licenses to merchants was important for maintaining the flow of goods into the city. But the commission was also willing to listen to and grant petitions from individuals who sought to move only private goods or personal property, and whose actions provided no larger public benefit. These were ordinary citizens who refused to allow the restrictions of the health commission to prevent them from continuing their lives, and who used their rights as citizens to petition the health commission, confident that they would be heard. By hearing and granting petitions, the health commission allowed many routines of travel and trade to continue, albeit at a slower pace, so it could work to limit the spread of plague without shutting down the city entirely. Thus, restrictions could be seen as effectively giving both the commission and residents a stronger sense of control.

The health commission received petitions from both men and women, from citizens able to compose their own petitions as well as those unable to sign their names, from merchants, monks, innkeepers, and householders, each of whom sought relief from restrictions. Most of the extant records are successful petitions, leaving unclear the extent to which any such petitions were unsuccessful. It is certainly possible that unsuccessful petitions were simply handled differently—recorded elsewhere or for some other reason not preserved. In any case, the remarkably large number of successful petitions demonstrates how effectively the system was utilized by both citizens and government. In the aggregate, the petitions preserved from each epidemic studied here (1582 and 1600) are uneven. There are far more individual petitions extant from 1582 than 1600, while there are more corporate petitions from the later epidemic, as city or town officials sought to renegotiate the quarantines imposed by officials in Seville. Taken together, they represent the voices of the people who lived through these epidemics and demonstrate the accessibility of municipal government.

The restrictions on what goods could be brought into the city could pose difficulties for residents in a variety of ways. For Juan Bautista, a resident of the city, the problem was his wife's dowry. Bautista married Juana de Vargava on a Sunday in late February 1582. Two days later, Bautista had to petition the health commission for permission to bring the furniture and clothing in his wife's dowry from the town where her family lived into the city where the couple was setting up household. As this meant passing through the city gates, Bautista needed the commission's permission to transfer the items. To this end, he presented two witnesses who each verified the facts of the case, testifying that they knew both bride and groom, that the two had just been married, and that they only wished to bring her dowry into the city. Satisfied, the commission granted Bautista his license the same day.[14] While the restrictions meant Bautista had to go to the additional trouble and effort of presenting a petition and lining up witnesses, his understanding of the routines of local government meant that his plans to set up a household in the city were unimpeded.

Other residents engaging in normal or expected routines could face similar difficulties. Both Esteban Martín and Isabel López sought at different times to move their respective households from outside the city walls to inside and faced resistance from gate guards. In both cases, testimonies from their parish priests affirming their health and the health of any other household members were sufficient to successfully gain entry for themselves and their personal belongings.[15] Wealthier households could face similar difficulties gaining entry for servants or slaves who had ventured outside the city for one reason or another. The tailor Manuel Pérez needed firsthand testimony from two acquaintances and a local doctor to persuade the council to allow his slave Pablo to reenter the city after a trip to Écija.[16] Isabel Guerrera's slave girl was stopped for carrying clothing with her, and was allowed to enter the city only after Guerrera had proved to the commission that it was her personal clothing the slave carried, and nothing else.[17] Doña Hortencia Vicéntelo likewise petitioned the commission on behalf of her servant, María de Senteno. According to Doña Hortencia, she had sent María on leave to visit her parents in the village of Zalamea, located about twenty-eight leagues outside the city. Upon asking María to return, Doña Hortencia learned that she was being detained in the village of Casaluenga because she did not carry any testimonies of health with her. Doña Hortencia provided the testimony of two other women to confirm the circumstances of María's travels and the reason for her lack of papers, successfully obtaining permission for María to come back into the city.[18]

Along with petitions for small individual requests, the commission heard many petitions from merchants seeking permission to import goods into the city. In 1582, for example, the epidemic was concentrated in the towns to the northeast of the city, an area that produced primarily wine and vinegar. Merchants like Diego de Escobar, accustomed to bringing wine from towns such as Constantina or Cazalla de la Sierra, suffered from their inability to continue to do so once plague had been declared in those towns. Of the individual petitions extant for four months in early 1582, nearly one-quarter (about 22 percent) are from wine merchants seeking permission to bring in varying quantities of wine. For nearly all these petitioners, the leprosy hospital of San Lazaro, located a distance outside the northern gates of the city, became a center for storage of goods awaiting inspection or quarantine.[19] A common requirement of the commission to such petitions was that wine had to not only sit for a period of quarantine, but also then had to be decanted into containers brought from the city and known to be clean, and transported into the city by local mules also known to be healthy. Merchants were generally willing to meet these requirements, and therefore could continue their trade.[20]

In March 1582, after helping to clear Gonzalo Martín to return home, the surgeon Bartolomé Hidalgo de Agüero confirmed the health of two other wine merchants, each of whom petitioned the health commission for permission to import a shipment of wine into the city. In each case, Hidalgo de Agüero also verified the health of the wine itself, as each shipment had spent a quarantine period sitting outside the city limits. The first of these merchants was Diego de Escobar, whose story of travels separate from his wine were recounted at the beginning of this chapter. The other was Clemente Muñoz.

Just four days after Gonzalo Martín had been removed from his house on suspicion he had come home from Constantina sick with plague, Clemente Muñoz asked for license to sell his wine in the city: "Clemente Muñoz resident of this city [of Seville] states that six days ago I brought seventy-four *arrobales* of wine from the town of Cazalla de la Sierra and having been ordered by your lordships not to allow entry to any people or goods from the town of Cazalla nor from the countryside around it, the guards would not let me enter."[21] Muñoz's petition prompted the health commission in Seville to increase efforts at quarantining Cazalla by ordering officials there to have their crier announce publicly that no persons whatsoever from the town would be allowed into Seville. This order specifically instructed that no clothing, wine, or other goods would be allowed entry either, and gave harsh penalties for disregarding the order, including four years in the galleys. Officials in Cazalla de la Sierra confirmed that they had received and made public these instructions just two days after Muñoz's petition.[22] Despite the commission's adamant stance against persons and wine from Cazalla de la Sierra, however, they did not turn Muñoz away. Instead, the commission ordered that the wine be decanted into barrels brought out from the city and held somewhere outside the city walls. Muñoz followed these instructions and stored his wine for over a month. It was early March when he appealed to the commission once again.[23] By this time, local officials in Cazalla had begun the process of lobbying the health commission to remove the restrictions for all of Cazalla's residents and goods, and the commission would be voting the next day to send a commissioner to investigate.[24] Muñoz, of course, had no way of knowing this and likely did not even know about the official attempts to lift the trade restrictions. In considering his second petition, in which Muñoz carefully pointed out the lengthy quarantine the wine had passed, the commission required further assurance that bringing the wine into the city would not pose any sort of health threat. This was when they again called on Bartolomé Hidalgo de Agüero to certify the health of the wine. Hidalgo de Agüero affirmed it to be healthy and safe, reporting that wine "cannot contain any contagion of pestilential and dangerous humors because it is a liquid and because the plague cannot be preserved except in textiles of linen or wool or silk."[25] Assured that the wine could not infect anyone, the commissioners granted Muñoz his license.

Later that same month, another local wine merchant, Benito Sánchez, likewise petitioned for permission to bring wine in for sale, but with fewer complications. Like Escobar, Sánchez explained to city officials how porters had carried his wine to the outskirts of town and stored it next to the hospital of San Lázaro. After waiting the requisite forty days, Sánchez then petitioned the health commission, offering several witnesses to prove that the wine had been brought to Seville the previous month, and had remained quarantined outside the city.[26]

In late April of 1582, in response to repeated entreaties from officials in Cazalla de la Sierra, the commission sent one of their own members to investigate that town's health. As a result of his positive report, the commission agreed to acknowledge Cazalla de la Sierra as now healthy and to lift the ban on its residents and goods. Several weeks later, however, the commission responded to new reports of plague and reimposed the ban. The day after the reimposition, the health commission heard four petitions from individuals, each claiming to be immediately in the process of bringing goods from Cazalla de la Sierra into the city when the new restrictions stopped them. A local woman, Marina Pérez, made the smallest request. She had sent to Cazalla de la Sierra for a small amount of vinegar for her own household and now needed official permission to receive it.[27] The largest request came from a local friar bringing in 250 *arrobales* of wine (approximately 1,065 gallons) for the College of Saint Thomas.[28] In addition, two other wine merchants each made a request, one to import 170 *arrobales* and the other 97 *arrobales* of wine (a combined total of approximately 1,137 gallons).[29] Willing to listen to merchants and ordinary residents alike, the health commission granted all four licenses.

One group for whom gate closures posed a particular problem was monks whose houses sat outside city walls. In the spring of 1600, for example, the health commission heard petitions from the priors of two monasteries, those of Nuestra Señora de los Remedios and Santísima Trinidad.[30] At the time, health officials had closed most of the city's gates to any traffic and each prior had the same request: that the city gate closest to their house be reopened for at least some hours each day. The prior of Santísima Trinidad even offered to provide monks as guards if the city so wished. Both houses had seen a precipitous drop in the offerings brought in by city residents who routinely visited the monasteries to pray in their chapels, hear mass, and be confessed. For both houses, such charitable and pious donations were a significant part of their income. In his petition, the prior of Nuestra Señora de los Remedios offered the city councilmen the choice of either opening the gate or providing financial support for the monastery themselves. In both cases, the health commission sent someone to investigate and report, and both gates were reopened for limited hours, guarded in one case by monks themselves (who received detailed instructions from the health commission) and in the other by municipally appointed guards.[31]

Similarly, the priests of San Vicente petitioned the council for the Royal Gate to be reopened with guards in order to give them access to the neighborhood known as Los Humeros. More than two hundred residents lived there, they claimed, all of them quite poor and often sick. Those in need of sacraments, especially those on their death beds, suffered greatly from the inability of the priests to reach them. The priests went as far as admitting to scaling the wall to reach their parishioners and hear confessions, but they could not easily transport the sacrament in so doing. After some consideration, the council granted their request, allowing them carry out their duties on both sides of city walls without further hindrance.[32]

Shipping and Trade

Throughout these years, Seville's port maintained steady traffic, despite the ongoing threat of plague. As a point of departure for the Indies fleets, the city maintained a constant flow of goods to be loaded onto the ships. In late April 1582, for example, Luís Ponce de León gained approval to bring 400 *arrobales* (1,074 gallons) of wine through the city in order to supply the fleet due to depart soon for New Spain.[33] In a reverse move, the city's plague commission granted permission in June 1600 for men to bring into the city goods salvaged from a ship in the Indies fleet. The ship had foundered on the sandbar at Sanlúcar de Barrameda, an all-too-frequent occurrence, and efforts to rescue reusable goods from it had hit their own impediment in the form of plague legislation. Anxious to save what they could, trade officials quickly appealed to city officials for permission to bring in the wine, vinegar, artillery, and armaments they had rescued. This was just one example of the competing authorities in the city (discussed in detail in chapter 5), but in this case city councilmen worked willingly with trade officials to give their approval, though city officials were still careful to forbid the entry of any mattresses or textiles from the ship.[34]

In addition, the port played a crucial part in Seville's role as a center of trade for both regional and international markets. The city housed a large community of resident foreign merchants who maintained an international network of trade and exchange.[35] This constant movement at port meant an additional area of concern for city officials wary of plague. Close quarters, poor diet, and unsanitary conditions meant sailors suffered a variety of frequent ailments, including various fevers; ships also had a notorious reputation for bringing hidden or unseen diseases into port, the motivation behind the development of the first quarantines at Ragusa.

n early April 1582, a Breton ship arrived at port in Seville with sick men board. The crew removed two dead sailors one morning, then that afternoon they moved another six who were sick to quarters on land. This was not tremendously unusual in and of itself, as sailors led hard lives, suffered a variety of ailments, and frequently died on board. But in times of plague, any death was noted with concern, so the health commission sent its clerk, Cristóbal Pérez, to investigate. Pérez began by checking with the local customs guards, and found only more rumors but no further details. Next, he interviewed two sailors from the ship. These men confirmed the deaths and illnesses, but disclaimed any dangerous illness (*ningun mal peligroso*), blaming instead fever and stomach disorders (*calentures y dolor de estomago*). Finally, he tracked down two physicians who had seen the sick men. The physicians confirmed that the illness was not contagious, asserting that they had found no evidence of swellings or buboes where they normally would appear on the body. This was sufficient to convince Pérez and the health commission that there was no danger from this ship.[36]

Nonetheless, additional precautions were put into effect to protect the city from foreign ships that might bring disease with them. Officials in the town of Coria del Río, located along the river just south of the city, were ordered to stop any vessels coming upriver that might have put in at any other port along the way. Many of the coastal areas, including the ports of Cádiz and Sanlúcar de Barrameda, were likewise suffering plague that year, and Seville's health commissioners were fearful of additional waves of disease being brought by ships that had visited those ports.[37] In order to bring goods into the city from the Atlantic, then, merchants in Seville sent orders to their ship captains to navigate upriver without stopping in any other port. Testimony that they had not stopped elsewhere became the key for obtaining permission to unload.

Anibal del Cacho, a Florentine living in Seville, petitioned the city council on May 4, 1582, for permission to unload a ship, the Santa María Buenaventura, which came from Italy loaded with various goods including paper, lace, and rice. In his initial petition, Cacho pointed out that the ship had departed from a clean port and had avoided both Cádiz and Sanlúcar as it came upriver. The council agreed to consider his petition and he returned the next day with the ship's notary, Honorato Brignole, and its captain, Alessandro Ferral. Both men gave detailed testimony on what the ship carried, where it had been, and that they had suffered no illnesses on board. They also presented the council with a letter, written in Italian, from the health officials of Villafranca. Dated March 17, the letter addressed the health officials in Cádiz and Seville, affirming the health of the ship as well as its captain, Alessandro Ferra. They also presented two brief testimonies of health from the city of Cartagena, dated April 2, where the ship had apparently first stopped. Three days later, on May 8, the council, having once again taken a professional consultation from Bartolomé Hidalgo de Agüero, who affirmed the health of all people and goods on the ship, agreed to allow for its unloading.[38]

Once again, this was not an unusual event. Within the first two weeks of May, an additional thirteen resident merchants requested permission to import a variety of goods for sale in the city, including wheat from Sicily, cloth from Flanders, paper from Italy, and wood from Galicia. Even while commissioners continued to investigate suspicious illnesses and deaths within the city itself, ships continued to arrive from abroad, their captains and crews little concerned over the possibility of contagion within the city. Provided they could show certificates of health from their home ports and provide witnesses to swear that the ships had not stopped in other ports, and that they could pass inspection by health commissioners looking for signs of pestilential fevers on board, those petitions were also granted.[39] Ships continued to arrive and unload, and much of the city's trade continued unabated.

Conflict

Despite the best intention of city councilmen, it was, of course, impossible to completely control the movements of all people and goods in and around the city. In part, this reflects the high degree of mobility of people in this era, often across quite large distances. In addition, it reflects the quick spread of news among officials in the various towns, including which areas were quarantined and which were not. Many travelers were stopped either at the city's gates or in surrounding towns. Those lacking travel papers most often claimed ignorance of the need for them (similarly claiming the town they started from was entirely healthy). Likewise, it was clearly a well-known tactic for travelers to simply travel first to a healthy town and pick up the necessary documentation of health. Diego de Escobar, whose efforts to bring wine into the city opened this chapter, had done so fairly easily. But he had also been entirely honest with everyone through this process, turning over to Seville's health commissioners all the related documents detailing his plan to gain papers by first visiting nonquarantined towns. Others were more cagey in their actions, seeking to gain papers under false pretense or not fully informing the commission of their prior movements.

The common restriction of closing or guarding city gates to restrict the inflow of people and goods was only effective for part of Seville. Of constant concern was the area where these restrictions couldn't work, the neighborhood of Triana. Separated from the rest of the city by the river, it had no walls encircling it, which made it easily accessible to visitors arriving along roads and paths that were difficult to monitor. Once in Triana, visitors could gain ready access to the main part of the city via river crossings that included both the wooden barge bridge and small ferry boats. In both 1582 and 1600, as in other epidemics, the councilmen repeatedly appointed individuals to patrol this area, monitoring both the roads themselves and any news circulating of travelers coming into town that way. In addition, councilmen in 1600 also ordered repairs to the *portillos* or smaller openings in the city walls that could allow unmonitored traffic into the city.[40] Those travelers without paperwork would be taken to the plague jail, located just outside the northernmost gate of the city (the Macarena gate).[41] Like the plague hospitals, the jail was a standard but not permanent feature in Seville by the sixteenth century. Located in houses or other buildings at the northern edge of town, in the neighborhood also known as La Macarena, the plague jail served as both quarantine station and holding station for those travelers either suspected of being ill or of circumventing the restrictions.[42]

The Guadalquivir River posed additional problems for health commissioners worried about monitoring travel. The river northward between Seville and Córdoba was dotted with small towns and river crossings, all of which allowed travelers easy movement from one side of the river to another. This perceived vulnerability prompted the health commission to pay particular attention to monitoring those other river crossings, in order to prevent travelers from taking a circuitous route to approach the city from the more open western edge.[43] Repeatedly in both epidemics, the health commissioners sent members to visit these river crossings either to instruct the ferrymen of their responsibility not to allow any travelers from certain towns passage across the river, or in some cases to assist in or oversee these restrictions. In early Februrary 1582, Diego de Toledo visited La Algaba, Cantillana, Tocina, Villanueva, and Alcalá del Río to instruct both town leaders and the local ferrymen of the dangers in giving passage to people from towns where plague had been declared.[44] In Alcalá del Río, Toledo instructed the ferryman to only allow passage to strangers if they first took their papers for approval to either the judge or another local councilman. By the end of the month, the commission in Seville had named councilmen to be posted in several of these towns to both oversee measures and assist in checking paperwork.[45]

Similarly, the health commission mandated that innkeepers in Seville were to refuse entry to any travelers without proper papers. In April 1600, this prompted a complaint from three innkeepers, Francisco González, Francisco Arenas, and Pedro Benítez, whose inns lay just outside city walls, but who were included in a requirement that any travelers wishing to stay there had to register with the closest gate guards, who would confirm their health and the paperwork they carried. Despite their pleas for exemption, as their patrons were people bringing supplies (*bastimentos*) into the city from the nearby countryside, the council reaffirmed these restrictions.[46]

Reports of known or suspected illegal entries into the city raised frequent investigations. In March 1582, two different commissioners, each working outside the city, sent news to the full commission of possible ways people were dodging restrictions. Juan de Perea, writing from Bodegón de las Cañas, warned that because the town of Carmona was not being guarded, travelers easily gained entrance then passed from there to Seville. Carmona lay on the other side of the Guadalquivir River from the towns then under quarantine (Constantina, Cazalla de la Sierra, La Puebla de los Infantes), and although guards checked travelers carefully at the river crossing of Tocina, Perea heard that many people from Constantina were said to cross the river just outside Tocina, passing thereby unchecked to Carmona and onward into the city.[47] The second commissioner, Diego de Toledo, wrote from the town of Alcalá del Río to warn the commission of two things. First, that he had spoken with a sheriff from the town of Fregenal who told him that the town of Castilblanco was heavily infected and suffering numerous deaths, though many people had left the town for the countryside. Second, he reported speaking with a councilman in Alcalá del Río who mentioned that on a visit to Seville a day previously, he had met several people from Castilblanco who were stopping at an inn in the neighborhood of Triana. Toledo put these pieces of information together and suggested that the commission check on this inn for cases of infection. Further, he advised that he had heard that a number of Moriscos from Castilblanco, carrying charcoal, had obtained false papers from nearby towns claiming health and now moved freely around Triana. As a result, he advised the commissioners not to take testimonies of health at face value, but rather to scrutinize them carefully.[48]

In other cases, travelers attempting to reach Seville found themselves stopped in the outlying towns, forced to argue their case to commissioners bent on preventing illegal entries. On March 14, 1582, Bernaldino Ramírez, a commissioner from Seville sent to monitor the town of La Rinconada and its outposts, stopped three suspicious travelers from Cazalla de la Sierra in the area of Casaluenga. The three identified themselves as Cristóbal Centeno, a lawyer; his sister María; and Juan de la Rosa, a tax collector. Questioned as to why they did not carry health papers with them, they informed Ramírez they were traveling on the orders of councilman Martín Santofímia Riquelme, who was then stationed in Cazalla de la Sierra, and that they carried letters from him to the *Asistente* and council in Seville. They requested permission to either continue on their journey or return to Cazalla, but Ramírez chose to detain them in the jail of La Rinconada, sending the letters onward and awaiting instructions from the Asistente. Two days later, the Asistente ordered them released to return to Cazalla de la Sierra.[49]

The same day, perhaps while Ramírez was occupied elsewhere dealing with the above case, his deputy, Francisco de Vergara, questioned two other men, Pedro González and Juan Esteban. González, a twenty-six-year-old shoemaker from the town of El Pedroso, had testimony with him but his companion Esteban did not. Upon interrogation, González easily admitted he had only met Juan Esteban recently while on the road from Cantillana to Seville. Esteban's travels had begun further north, in the town of Azuaga, which lay outside of Seville's jurisdiction. As Vergara took this testimony, two additional travelers appeared, declaring themselves Esteban's companions. Alonso Gallego and Santiago Rubio, also from Azuaga, testified that they were heading to Seville to try and negotiate passage to the New World. They had heard along the way that plague had broken out and several towns were being monitored, but they decided to continue onward. Each man testified that he did not carry any papers with him because he didn't realize that they were necessary. Esteban also swore that he had joined Pedro González simply because they met up on the road, but he had not attempted to slip past authorities on the basis of González's papers, nor had he bribed González into letting him tag along on his credentials. Vergara ordered Estevan, Gallego, and Rubio jailed and fined for traveling without proper documents, then turned the case over to Bernaldino Ramírez. Ramírez in turn sent the case to the Asistente in Seville, who ordered the three transported under guard to Seville's plague jail.[50]

Within days, the commission in Seville received testimony regarding another case of travelers with questionable papers, this time from Diego de Toledo, who was in the town of Alcalá del Río. Four muleteers transporting a large quantity of wine had appeared in the town on the evening of March 18, claiming to have arrived from the town of Cabeza de Vaca. Although they carried papers from Cabeza, those papers made no reference of where these men resided (where they were *vecinos*), which raised Toledo's suspicions. In addition, the men traveled with a young boy, not mentioned in any of their papers. Toledo interviewed the boy, named Tomás, who gave him two letters he carried to Seville. The letters confirmed Toledo's suspicion. Written by the boy's father in Segura de León, they detailed the deaths of family members due to plague.[51] The boy's father had arranged for Tomás to travel with the muleteers to Seville to find his older brother Juan, who had previously traveled there in the same way. Carefully interviewing each of the men, then, Toledo found that they in fact were originally from Segura de León, and had been advised to carry a load first to Cabeza de Vaca in order to obtain travel papers from a notary there.[52] After taking all this testimony, Toledo appealed to the commission and *Asistente* for permission to detain the men and burn the clothing they carried with them, though it was "little."[53] In the end, the Asistente permitted the wine to be sent onward to the city, provided it was transported in skins brought from the city, but the men and young Tomás were to return to Segura de León.[54]

In other cases, travelers aroused official suspicion simply by virtue of their movements, but were not arrested. Such was the case in early February 1582,

...ion sent Alonso Rodríguez and the comm...
...o check up on two women who had recently a...
...n of Constantina.[55] The women, later identifie...
...Ana Martín, had apparently come to visit relatives i...
...ity prior to the restrictions against travelers from tha...
which we... posed at the end of January. They stayed first in Triana, crossed the river after a week to find Juana de Llerena's daughter, in ... *corral*, or tenement, where she lived. It was then that the health commi... sion learned of the women's presence in the city. The commission ordered Rodríguez and Pérez to find the women, discover whether either of them was sick, and, if so, to call a physician. In addition, the men were to find out whether the two women had brought any textiles with them, which would be subject to confiscation and either burning or isolation in the countryside.[56]

Arriving at the *corral*, the men found that the women had left. So they instead interviewed three female residents of the *corral*, each of whom testified under oath to what little they knew of Llerena and Martín. The fourth witness they interviewed was Juana de Llerena's daughter, also named Juana. She confirmed the visit of her mother and a friend, filling in some missing details. The two women had indeed come from Constantina, arriving first in Triana to stay a week with Juana's sister Francisca Martín. They had then spent two weeks with Juana, then left to go separate ways. Juana de Llerena was returning to her other daughter's house, while Ana Martín planned to visit unnamed friends or relatives elsewhere in the city.[57] The two men followed up on this testimony the next day, visiting the house in Triana where Francisca Martín lived and worked as a servant. Unable to speak with Francisca directly, they spoke instead with her employer, Inés de Plata, who confirmed Juana de Llerena's visit and testified that she was healthy.[58]

The commissioners made a deliberate public show of investigating, taking testimony and following up on it. Yet two days of investigation had turned up little more than a chain of testimony about two women who were never located. All of the women asked to testify concerning Juana and Ana had confirmed their health and that they brought no goods, especially textiles, with them. While the actions of the commissioners in this case amounted to no real results, and perhaps seem a waste of time and energy, they may also be read as an important public display of official action, both assuring and warning the community of the seriousness with which they enforced plague restrictions. Seen from the point of view of health officials, the arrival and movement of these women would have been suspicious. By arriving first in Triana, the two women gained access to the city through the least protected quarter. Their movements, seemingly one step ahead of the officials investigating them, could only have enhanced suspicion surrounding them. Yet officials in this case were not relentless. They followed all leads, spoke with everyone they found who had contact with the women, but willingly stopped

ation without ever seeing or directly addressing the wo..
Their objectives had been met through the course of their inter·
y had alerted all those residents who had contact with the women
ossible health threat they could pose and had received testimony in
that Llerena and Martín were by all accounts healthy and innocent of
ts to evade officials. Most important, health officials had made known
ir presence and interest in tracking down possible health threats.

Health commissioners in Seville worked in a seemingly endless cycle of
petitions and investigations, trying to balance potential public health risks
against potential economic risks. The system of health passports or papers
was certainly not foolproof, but it was the best system they had for gaining
some sense of control over a mobile population. Commissioners tempered
their authority by balancing cautious leniency in some cases with strict
enforcement in others. Sorting through the cacophony of opinions, pleas,
demands, and advice, commissioners made the best decisions they could to
keep the city running with as little scandal or disruption as possible. Assisted,
for the most part, by a populace willing to play by the rules, they nonetheless watched carefully for those attempting to break them. All the while, a
similar tableau of restriction, petition, and exemption played out at a larger
regional level as officials in Seville interacted continuously not only with
their own investigating commissioners but also with officials from numerous
other cities working to negotiate the imposition and removal of travel bans.

Chapter Four

The Wider Politics of Public Health

Balancing Urban and Rural

Plague commissioners remained highly visible as they maintained contact with large numbers of residents, moving around the city to follow up on petitions, inspect goods, and check up on the sick. Amid this flurry of activity, a number of commissioners were also sent outside the city to carry out many of the same activities in the towns and villages of the tierra. They did so not just in the interest of protecting the city's residents, but also in the interest of all residents within the tierra. Monitoring the movement of people and goods around the countryside allowed commissioners to provide warnings and protective measures in areas before plague broke out. This meant that rather than creating isolation and limiting communication between cities and towns, in many cases plague actually increased official contact and communication.

Like all early modern cities, Seville engaged in a network of trade both locally, within its tierra, and regionally, across Andalucía. In addition, Seville's unique position as trade center for the New World made it all the more imperative for the city council to facilitate the continued operation of these trade networks. Yet the effects of plague legislation could range from disruptive to disastrous. Historians have long seen the negative effects of these bans as trade dwindled and travel became difficult. In his demographic study of early modern Cuenca, David Reher asserts that "the appearance or the mere rumor of disease had disastrous effects on the local economy. Efforts to isolate the town brought commercial activities to a halt, created a shortage of labor, stimulated inflation and otherwise tended to undermine most economic activity."[1] Similarly, Linda Martz, examining poverty in early modern Toledo, describes "plague restrictions that prohibited the movement of merchandise and people" as one of the many disasters that could push merchants or peasants into poverty.[2] Such economic problems are shown in a variety of records from cities across Spain. Yet there was another side here also. Plague certainly disrupted trade, prompting the health commission to effectively shut trade routes down. And when this happened, the economic balance was lost, and subsistence crises were often created. As Francisco Perellón reported from Constantina in early 1582, the increase in plague there had prompted many residents to flee to their farmlands for fear of the lack of provisions.[3] But just as individuals within the city worked with plague commissioners to restore a necessary balance, both the towns within Seville's tierra and cities more distant from Seville took a similar initiative to communicate with one another, sending letters and emissaries back and forth until a new balance could be reached between the sometimes opposing needs of economics and public health. In this way, epidemics of the sixteenth century may serve to illuminate two important aspects of life in early modern Spain. Epidemics (and the responses to them) shed light on the deep integration of both societies and economies of city and town in early modern Spain.[4] For many towns, and certainly for a central city such as Seville, the heroic self-isolation for which the English town of Eyam is still justly famous simply wasn't possible.[5] In addition, the actions and movements of Seville's plague commissioners offer further insight into the peculiar balance of medical beliefs that encouraged civic leaders to continue their work without fear or hesitation, thereby enabling these societies to maintain their integration.

Investigations

In the town of Constantina 18 January 1582 the excellent gentleman Juan de Perea Durán, judge commissioned by his excellency the Count, governor of the city and territory of Seville . . . in the presence of myself, the clerk, stated that it has come to his attention that the town of Cazalla de la Sierra is infected with a contagion, which is the cause of the present commission.[6]

When Seville's city council first took note of the impending contagion in 1582, it was because of unofficial news that plague was breaking out in the town of Cazalla de la Sierra. In response, Seville's councilmen sent Juan de Perea Durán, a judge in the town of La Puebla de los Infantes, to the neighboring town of Constantina, along with a surgeon, Pedro García Arroyal. The two arrived in Constantina on January 18 and immediately set to work taking testimony from residents.[7] In this case, Perea Durán was investigating rumors of plague, not in the town he was visiting (Constantina), but in the neighboring town of Cazalla de la Sierra. So he began with the source of news from Cazalla de la Sierra, a local innkeeper. The innkeeper testified that he had overheard Andrés Hernández, son of Diego Hernández, say that a barber by the name of Juan del Barco had died, along with his wife and children, in the town of Cazalla de la Sierra. The younger Hernández presumably knew this firsthand, as he had returned from Cazalla de la Sierra just the day before. Upon hearing this news, the innkeeper wrote to his brother-in-law, Francisco Gutiérrez, also resident in Cazalla. In response, Gutiérrez confirmed the deaths of the del Barco family. Gutiérrez also informed him that his own son had also been ill with plague, manifested by a bubo behind the ear. Happily, he reported, the boy recovered from his illness after treatment by both a barber-surgeon and a physician.[8]

Following these accounts, Perea Durán took sworn testimony from two other men, Andrés Hernández himself, and Luis de Andraza, the sheriff (*alguacil executor*) of Constantina, who had also recently been visiting Cazalla de la Sierra. Hernández, a young man of twenty, confirmed that he had been in Cazalla the day before and had heard of the deaths of six people in one house, but that this was all he knew. Andraza supplemented the rumors with further evidence, testifying that he had been in Cazalla on the 14th of January and saw a young girl carried to the church there. Upon asking, he was told that she had been healthy and well fed, but had died after only five days, apparently of the plague. Andraza had then asked the vicar about recent illnesses and was told that four people had died recently, which the vicar understood to all be from plague (*landres*). Another local woman told Andraza that at least one house had been boarded up because of plague deaths there.[9]

Juan de Perea Durán's only real job in Constantina was to collect information, to act as eyes and ears for the health commission in Seville. After copying the testimony of all three men and sending it to Seville's health commission, he continued his efforts in the town until relieved five days later by Diego de Toledo, a health commissioner sent directly from Seville. Upon reading and evaluating the information supplied by Perea Durán, the city council in Seville had named a new plague commission, whose first action was to send Toledo to replace him. This allowed Perea Durán to return to La Puebla de los Infantes, which by then was also beginning to experience suspicious deaths. Perea Durán returned to La Puebla accompanied again by the surgeon Pedro García Arroyal.[10]

Commissioners like Toledo working outside of the city had, in many ways, a heavier task on their hands than those remaining in the city. They were individually responsible for coordinating the precautions and sanitary measures of an entire town or village. While the commission as a whole made many of the important decisions regarding any municipality, the commissioners were still locally responsible for implementing them. Above all, however, the commissioners gathered and reported information. They did so with the same attention to detail and precision of the commissioners working within the city. Diego de Toledo and the other commissioners reported not only on medical information such as the number sick, dead, and recovering, and the state of the local medical resources, which included the supply of necessary provisions, but also on the current price of wheat, and even the moods or emotions of town residents. In all the towns he visited, Toledo followed the same course of action, repeatedly issuing reports that quickly become rather tediously redundant. What is remarkable about them is not so much what he did, as the frequency with which he did it, and the diligence with which he carried out his routine of detailed investigation and recording over and over.

In early 1582, at the same time that the wine merchant Diego de Escobar began his process of travel and petition, town leaders in Cazalla de la Sierra began a process of a corporate petition from the town as a whole to be removed from the list of infected towns. In the words of one petitioner, the surgeon Andrés Gutiérrez, "the greater hardship of the people is starvation, for the foodstuffs that they are accustomed to living on are no longer brought into the town."[11] Had Seville's health commission simply enacted and then rigidly enforced their restrictions, Cazalla's residents would indeed have suffered and the town might well have become the "gruesome pastiche of hell" described by Brockliss and Jones. Instead, the health commission worked to monitor the health situation and precautions being taken in banned towns, often by sending a plague commissioner to collect information firsthand and report back.

The commissioners working to investigate plague met with both resistance and welcome. A commissioner who found no sickness or suspicious deaths in a town could prevent the imposition of a quarantine. If he did find reason for caution or quarantine, a plea from the commissioner would go a long way toward getting the town monetary, medical, or other assistance.[12] For the people experiencing an epidemic, or concerned at the threat of one, the commissioners could be an unwelcome and disruptive intrusion into their lives and daily routines, but they could also represent people's best hope to resume those routines once they had been disrupted. On the one hand, if the commissioners believed plague to have infected a household, they could order people or families removed from the city, their clothing and bedding burned. Their findings of plague led to the quarantining of towns, disrupting the normal flow of trade. Such intrusions and disruptions certainly prompted efforts to evade authorities by hiding the sick or claiming other causes of death. On the other hand, the commissioners offered official action and the hope of relief. For just as they could impose a diagnosis of plague and subsequent restrictions on a person or entire town, they also held the power to lift that diagnosis and the resultant restrictions. Visiting commissioners gave the townspeople a chance to present their side—to show that if some were sick, not all were, and how well the town had things under control. If the epidemic was indeed raging in the town, the visiting commissioner could become an advocate for local residents, requesting supplies, money, or even additional medical personnel.[13] In addition, the presence of a commissioner, particularly when there were suspicious or worrisome deaths in a town, could be a calming influence. Rather than just an ominous presence, a commissioner was also a link to higher powers (that is, the commission and the city council), and therefore to assistance and relief. He could give people a sense that action was being taken, that they were being listened to and the information was being recorded, and most important, that they were not simply at the mercy of the epidemic.

The constant contact of Diego de Toledo and other mobile commissioners with residents of infected towns is another sign of the multiple and varying beliefs regarding disease causation in this era. The very willingness of city officials to continually visit towns believed infected with plague reflects their belief that they themselves were not at risk. Sent repeatedly away from home, none of the commissioners made any effort to shirk their duties or to avoid any towns or individuals, displaying no fear of being in proximity to the very people and places most likely infected. While the official response to plague still relied heavily on isolation or avoidance of the sick, officials themselves traveled rather easily in and out of the city, moving around the infected countryside without hesitation. None mention any preventive measures they themselves may have taken (such as using masks or handkerchiefs to cover their nose and mouth to keep miasmatic air out), though they record other details of their work. And while commissioners did not generally have contact with the sick themselves, they were in constant contact with those involved in patient care: physicians, apothecaries, priests. Here again, continual references in their reports to poverty and lack of wholesome food reflect their likely belief that they were protected by their status, lifestyle, and diet. In any case, their actions present an intriguing alternative to the traditional view of fear, rejection, and abandonment as standard responses to plague.

At times commissioners like Diego de Toledo played a dual role. They represented the government in Seville, but became advocates of the towns they found healthy. While some reports were simple listings of the ill and dead, others reveal a more human side to the crisis, such as Diego de Toledo's report of the happiness of a young girl upon her release from the hospital in Constantina.[14] Commissioners were not simply detached observers. Shortly after returning to La Puebla, Juan de Perea Durán related having heard news of a woman who had fled from La Puebla six days previously for the city of Córdoba, and had subsequently died there, perhaps a warning of the direction the epidemic was spreading. But the last part of his letter is a plea to help the residents of La Puebla, pointing out that since the commission has ordered residents not be allowed to leave, they are dying of starvation for not being able to go out to work their lands.[15]

While Perea Durán reported all this to the commission in Seville, Diego de Toledo set to work in Constantina, taking charge of the town's epidemic response and preparedness. He sent the commission several reports, each dated January 20. While Toledo makes no reference to the fact that this was he feast day of St. Sebastian, patron saint of plague, such an irony would surely not have been lost on those receiving his letters. The first was a general report of the state of the town, which he found subdued but mostly healthy. Of the eight plague patients then held in the local hospital, "two have died and four of the six are in good disposition."[16] Along with this overview of the town, Toledo sent an account of his inspection of the town's pharmacy and the inventory of twenty-two ingredients stocked by pharmacist Pedro Ramírez. He called on a local doctor to inspect them and affirm their freshness. The final two documents Toledo sent were an account of his discussion with local officials regarding money collected and paid during this epidemic and an account of having commissioned a local judge, Francisco Perellón, to take charge of health matters on behalf of the city's health commission. Toledo finished his business in Constantina in just three days, after which he moved on to spend a day in the town of La Puebla de los Infantes, and then returned to Seville to follow up his written reports with his own testimony and receive new instructions.[17]

Diego de Toledo serves as a good example of a hardworking plague commissioner. He was an active and respected member of the city council for many years. Not only did he work tirelessly during the epidemic of 1582, but he may also be found still hard at work in the council at the outbreak of the next widespread epidemic in 1599.[18] He seems to have been one of the busiest commissioners during the 1582 epidemic, or at least the most well-traveled. In the five months of January to May, Toledo made nineteen trips to eleven different outlying towns (see table 4.1), generally traveling back to Seville for a period of days before heading out again, though sometimes visiting two or even three towns in one trip. Despite his extensive and almost continuous travels, Toledo made no mention of his extraordinary efforts. Only in systematically searching the accounts of the health commission can they be pieced together.

Diego de Toledo was far from the only commissioner working outside the city. In this same epidemic, numerous other commissioners were sent out on similar missions, helping the commission coordinate and manage the city's response to the growing epidemic. Although still active in the city council in 1599, Toledo no longer traveled as he had earlier. Other, presumably younger and heartier commissioners took over the duties of traveling, such as Alonso Leandro de Herrera, some of whose movements in the months of March and April 1600 are shown in table 4.2.

For most of these travels, Herrera likewise carried out a routine of notification. He traveled where he was sent, carrying with him letters from the council announcing the confirmed infection of the town of Morón and requesting cooperation from local officials in monitoring and screening travelers.[19] An exception to this routine came in late April, on his visit to Granada, which is detailed below. In that case, Herrera had been named by

Table 4.1. Diego de Toledo's travels in 1582

January 18	Constantina
February 8	La Algaba
February 8	Alcalá del Río
February 8	La Puebla de los Infantes
February 12	Cantillana
February 13	Lora
February 13	Tocina
February 14	Alcalá del Río
February 14	Villanueva
February 14	Alcolea
February 15	Tocina
February 18	Sevilla
February 20	Alcolea
February 22	Sevilla
February 24	Alcalá del Río
February 26	Sevilla
February 28– March 27	Alcalá del Río
March 29	Sevilla
April 9	Alcalá del Río
April 16	Coria
April 20	Sevilla
April 20	Alcalá del Río
April 21	Sevilla
April 26	Coria
May 4	Sevilla

Source: AMS, sección 13, siglo XVI, tomos 5, 6.

Table 4.2. Alonso Leandro de Herrera's travels in 1600

March 17–18	Utrera
March 20	Alcalá de Guadaira
March 21	Seville
March 30	Villafranca
April 1	Lebrija
Before April 10	Las Cabezas de San Juan
April 16–20	Granada

Source: AMS, sección 7, tomo 7, no. 17.

the council to investigate the health status of the city, not just to notify officials of other infected towns.

Commissioners like Diego de Toledo and Alonso Leandro de Herrera represented only one part of a larger system of information collection. Also contributing information on the health of towns were local officials and doctors. Juan de Perea Durán, for example, sent regular updates from La Puebla de los Infantes to the health commission in Seville during the epidemic of 1582, while in the town of Constantina, Dr. Centurio kept the commission updated on the numbers of illnesses until his own death at the end of March. His replacement, Miguel Díaz, was appointed shortly thereafter by the health commission and soon picked up the task of reporting on the town's health.[20]

Networks of Communication

Throughout the epidemic of 1582, Seville's council was in correspondence, either sporadically or continuously, with twenty-five neighboring towns. In the 1599–1600 epidemic, which was far more widespread, the commission maintained correspondence with over forty towns and cities, some as far away as Granada (see table 4.3). The commission thus functioned as a center of information and communication for the entire territory.

As discussed above, when doctors or residents reported cases of plague in these outlying towns, the city responded by first sending a commissioner to confirm the outbreak, then placing the infected town under a general quarantine. This meant formally forbidding residents or goods entry into the city (with both a public announcement and the addition of the town's name to a list maintained on public notice boards). In addition, the city would send notices to neighboring towns, or those towns that lay on travel routes between the infected town and Seville, alerting them to the quarantine and advising similar measures. In reaction to such municipal quarantines, individuals such as Diego de Escobar could and did petition for individual relief. But the town leaders themselves had a similar recourse and the city's health commission was just as willing to entertain corporate petitions as individual ones.

In the sixteenth century, the many large and small towns that made up Seville's tierra depended heavily on one another both socially and economically. The city depended on the towns of its tierra to provide agricultural resources. The towns themselves maintained specialized production and relatively small food stores for times of crisis. Cazalla de la Sierra, Constantina, and other nearby towns were well-known for the wine and vinegar they produced, while towns in other parts of Seville's tierra produced wheat, onions, charcoal, and other products.[21] Once a town lost its ability to trade freely, it could quickly face a subsistence crisis, which made it urgent to negotiate

Table 4.3. Towns within Seville's tierra in communication with plague commission

1582	1599–1600
Alcalá del Río	Acufre
Alcolea del Río	Alanís
Bodegón de las Cañas	Alcalá de Guadaira
Bodonal	Aracena
Burguillos	Aroche
Cantillana	Bodonal
Casaluenga	Cala
Castilblanco	Carmona
Cazalla de la Sierra	Castilblanco
Constantina	Castillo de las Guardas
Cumbres de San Bartolomé	Cazalla de la Sierra
El Garrobo	Constantina
Encinasola	Coronel
Fregenal de la Sierra	Cortegana
Guadalcanal	Cumbres de San Bartolomé
La Algaba	Cumbres en medio
La Puebla de los Infantes	Cumbres mayores
Lora	El Almadén
Peñaflor	El Cerro
La Rinconada	El Garrobo
San Isidro del Campo	El Pedroso
Santiponce	El Real de la Jara
Segura de León	Encinasola
Tocina	Fregenal de la Sierra
Valdepeñas	Galaroza
Villanueva del Río	Higuera de Aracena
	Higuera de Fregenal
	Hinojales
	La Marotera
	La Nava
	La Puebla de los Infantes
	Las Cabezas de San Juan
	Lebrija
	Morón de la Frontera
	Paterna
	Santa Olalla del Cala
	Utrera
	Villafranca

Source: AMS, sección 13, tomas 5, 6; sección 7, tomo 7, no. 17.

a reopening of trade. In addition, towns and villages were the population centers for farmlands that surrounded them, so strict quarantine measures could even impinge on residents' willingness or ability to leave town to work their holdings and regain entry to their homes.[22]

In the 1582 epidemic, the list of infected towns continued to grow—first Cazalla de la Sierra, then La Puebla de los Infantes, then Constantina and later Jerez, which lay to the north of Seville near the city of Badajoz. The geographic distinction, "near Badajoz," was used in all references to the town to distinguish it from Jerez de la Frontera, the more widely known town southwest of Seville, whose name the English had anglicized to denote its famous export, sherry. Within a month, the health commission in Seville began to take measures designed to create a buffer zone of protection between the infected towns to the northeast and the city proper. In late February, the plague commission ordered five of its members to the towns of San Isidro del Campo, El Garrobo, Casaluenga, Villanueva del Río, and Alcalá del Río, all of which lay along the travel routes between the infected towns and the city.[23] Each commissioner traveled with two deputies, carrying with them official proclamations of infection in the four towns, as well as orders to oversee all the necessary precautions in the uninfected towns to prevent the contagion from entering. Primarily, this meant setting up guards at town gates and river crossings. Any persons traveling from the direction of these infected towns had to state their business, and had to produce an official testimony stating the town of their origin and the health of that town. In doing so, the health commission hoped to prevent the spread of plague to uninfected towns, but more important, they wanted to set up an extra layer of protection for the city, a local cordon sanitaire. Without intending to, however, the health commission created a municipal quarantine that imperiled the infected towns by removing them from their normal routines of trade with both the city and all surrounding towns. It is this predicament that has most often been pointed out by historians asserting the dire consequences of plague epidemics. By examining the situation of Cazalla de la Sierra in closer detail, however, we can see a slightly different picture.

Cazalla de la Sierra serves as a good sample town for exploring relations between city and countryside in part because it suffered a great deal during the epidemic of 1582. Because of this, officials in Cazalla were in frequent communication with their counterparts in Seville, generating a large number of petitions and testimonies that can help shed light on how towns negotiated with the municipal health commission. Located approximately twelve leagues (forty-one miles) to the northeast of Seville, Cazalla de la Sierra had roughly two thousand residents.[24] It was one of the first towns to report suspicious deaths in 1582, although it was one of the last to be visited by a health commissioner. As discussed above, rumors of plague in Cazalla de la Sierra in late January had prompted the city council to send first Juan de

Perea Durán, and later Diego de Toledo, to the town of Constantina where the news had originated. Toledo's report to the commission prompted them to declare both towns infected.

In Cazalla de la Sierra, local leaders began by sending a letter to the city council, dated February 8, confirming that they had received the news declaring their people and goods infected. The letter acknowledged the restrictions and carefully restated the penalties to be imposed for breaking these restrictions: for the wealthy, a fine of 100,000 *maravedís* and four years in the galleys without wages; for poorer folk, the fine was replaced by two hundred lashes and the same four years in the galleys. They followed up by sending sworn testimony from the town crier that he had announced the restrictions and penalties in the town square. This was the first step to renegotiating relations with the city—the acknowledgment of the city's restrictions and assurances given back that the town was doing all that it could to comply with them, as well as a recounting of other measures to contain the spread of plague.[25]

Local authorities, led by the town judge, then followed up a week later by sending the city council an appeal for relief from the quarantine. They compiled sworn testimony from thirteen local doctors, surgeons, and clerics; those who were in the best position to affirm whether or not anyone in town was sick.[26] In their testimonies these men all emphatically repeated the same message over and over: that the town, though previously suffering plague, was now healthy, no new cases of illness had developed, and that the real threat to survival was starvation and the need for food. As it was these local officials who had taken the initiative of communicating with Seville's health commission, their initial testimonies emphasized what was most important to them: the lack of provisions. Each of the witnesses asserted that the threat of the disease had died down, but now the threat was the lack of provisions "by which they are accustomed to sustaining themselves," a breakdown in the reciprocity of trade that provided foodstuffs for the people of the town. These testimonies are highly formulaic and repetitive, masking objective assessment of health behind persuasive statements that downplayed the issue of illness but emphasized instead that of the need for provisions.

Seville's council responded by monitoring the situation, but quietly. They voted on February 22 to send a secret representative to investigate the health of the town, and received his report by March 2.[27] But because there had been no public response from Seville's council, the authorities in Cazalla waited a short time, then decided to try again. They collected a second set of testimonies, this time from nineteen men.[28] This second set, dated February 26, included not only many of the same men who had testified in the previous appeal, but also several wealthy and important local men, such as Enrique de Guzmán Ponce de León. Their testimony was taken not because they had any expertise or medical knowledge, but rather because as members of the upper class, they were presumed to be highly credible. In addition, local nobles were the most likely to have the means and inclination to leave town in the face of danger, and as Guzmán himself pointed out, had there been any health danger, he and others would have removed themselves to live elsewhere. This can be seen in the later epidemic of 1600, when the Duke of Medina Sidonia first sent his wife out of Seville to stay with relatives, then later joined her as the epidemic expanded within the city.[29] This second appeal from Cazalla is markedly different from the first in another way. The first set of testimonies all mention that the town had indeed been suffering from an epidemic but the danger was now over. Here, the town leaders focused on the plague commission's greatest concern, the health of the town. The second set of testimonies does not even mention the town's earlier cases of plague. Instead, the formula now changed to each person emphasizing that the town was not just healthy, but healthier than in it had been in years. In the words again of Andrés Gutiérrez, "this town and its residents are free of any plague or other contagious disease and that not one person has died of these maladies and that by the grace of God, so little illness has never been seen in this town."[30] Here is clearly some rhetorical exaggeration, which was common in this era. Yet, it should be noted, not all official accounts were always so positive in the face they presented. The first set of testimonies contained admissions from doctors that they still treated a number of fevers and other maladies at the time. In addition, as we'll see later, doctors readily admitted when plague did seem to have broken out again.

That the officials in Cazalla remained concerned about their lack of provisions is evident in the cover letter that accompanied this second petition. In this way, the town presented its needs to the city in a brief letter, then backed up its request for relief with numerous testimonies that repeatedly assured that the town was healthy. Seville's plague commission could not ignore such a plea. By this time, it had also received a report from Hernan Carillo de Saavedra, who affirmed that his secret inquiries had shown no illness in Cazalla, only hunger. In response, the commission made a more public display of investigating, naming Martín de Santofímia Riquelme to visit and gather evidence.[31]

Allotted eight days for his investigation, but also ordered to maintain secrecy, Riquelme quickly set to work upon his arrival in Cazalla two days later.[32] There was little secret about Riquelme's movements, however, as he went about the town interviewing, investigating, following up. He began by visiting the hospital and its six patients. The local doctor, Hernando Vázquez, accompanied Riquelme as he visited each patient, giving the diagnosis for each: two suffering "pain in their side" (*dolor de costado*), one from fever (*unos calenturas*), one woman suffering dropsy (*una muger ydropica*), and the remaining two recovering from other unspecified fevers (*calenturas*).

Riquelme then took a formal deposition from the doctor, who swore that he had treated a number of cases of plague at the end of January that year, but most had recovered successfully. According to Doctor Vázquez, there had been no cases of plague for the past twenty days and the town was over-all very healthy.[33] Other medical figures Riquelme interviewed agreed with Vázquez that the town was then healthy, though they did not agree on the extent of plague in previous months. Where Vázquez downplayed the earlier epidemic, saying he had treated a few cases, of which only three or four had died, others who Riquelme interviewed agreed that in total some forty or fifty people had died in the epidemic that began around Christmastime and continued into early February.[34] Later that same day, Riquelme observed the priest at the town's main church taking the sacrament to a house-bound parishioner. He quickly sent one of his assistants to find out where the priest was going and why. Learning that the householder, Fulano Ortega, was too ill to attend church services, Riquelme again turned to Doctor Vázquez, who reported that Ortega was his patient and did not have plague.[35] In the course of his investigation, Riquelme visited two local pharmacists and the jail, interviewed doctors, surgeons, pharmacists, clergy, and various residents. While he was in Cazalla de la Sierra, three residents died. Riquelme checked on each death, carefully watching for any signs that plague was still lurking somewhere in the town, ready to burst forth again. His final report to the health commission was thirty-one pages long, a thorough accounting of all interviews he conducted, deaths he investigated, and preventive measures he enforced. Everyone he spoke with confirmed that there had not been any plague deaths in the town for over twenty days, and so little sickness had never before been observed. His visit ended with a celebration in the town and thanksgiving for health in the form of a religious procession by the town's brotherhoods and con-fraternities.[36] His report to the cabildo found that the town, while perhaps not experiencing "fewer illnesses than ever before" as the town's doctors had asserted, was generally healthy. As a result, restrictions against trade with the town were lifted at the end of March, and citizens of Cazalla were once again allowed free entry to Seville.[37]

Towns that traditionally enjoyed a close relationship with the city reserved the right to negotiate when that relationship changed. And this was a pro-cess of negotiation, for just as it imposed them, the commission could and did rescind restrictions and reopen trade and other relations, once it was presented with what it considered sufficient evidence that the possibility of contagion had passed. At the same time, the commission had the power and was willing to grant individual petitions for special permission to enter the city or to use certain city gates, again when presented with persuasive evi-dence of necessity and safety. The commission did not wield its power capri-ciously. Its restrictions were not arbitrary, but were agreed on by consensus after an investigation. In many cases, the restrictions simply opened a process of negotiation as both individuals and municipalities sought to alter the terms. It is ironic that for many towns, the crisis of an epidemic brought about a dramatic increase in official contact and communication with the city at the same time that a quarantine limited individual contact.

Cazalla de la Sierra's citizens enjoyed a brief resumption of normal life, including access to the city, before plague broke out once again. A month after they lifted the original ban, Seville's health commission reimposed a quarantine on April 25.[38] Such a shift from infected to healthy, then back to infected, raises the question of why the quarantine was lifted at all. There is no clear answer in the extant records, but there is good reason to infer that Seville's plague commission was attempting to balance a variety of concerns. Pestilential diseases were highly variable and notoriously difficult to predict as they could quickly wax and wane. So when all the information, including Riquelme's extensive report, seemed to indicate that the threat of plague had passed, it made sense to reopen trade. Only when the death rates suddenly jumped again did new restrictions become unavoidable for the larger common good.

As discussed previously, the new restrictions against Cazalla caught several people off guard. The very next day, the council heard from petitions from three people, each of whom was in the process of bringing wine or vinegar from Cazalla into the city.[39] Indeed, one petitioner claimed that he was bringing his wine to the Macarena gate just at the exact moment he heard the proclamation read, quite an unhappy coincidence.[40] The commission clearly saw little point in denying these individuals the right to complete their transactions, and the benefits to both the individuals and the city outweighed the risks. As hurtful as the municipal quarantines were to the outlying towns, they also limited the city's access to provisions and the ability of some local merchants to earn a living.

Following the recondemnation of Cazalla de la Sierra at the end of April, the plague commission sent yet another representative to investigate. On May 7, Ambrosio Ramírez de Sierra arrived in Cazalla and prepared to spend a number of days collecting information. He questioned many of the same local doctors, pharmacists, and other officials as the previous commissioner, but this time the message was not so optimistic. It seemed that the town had indeed been suffering plague for the past month, though the worst appeared once again to be over. The report compiled by Ramírez contained an extraordinary amount of detail, as each person questioned recounted not only the numbers of ill, but also the names of all local residents who had fallen sick or died during the most recent epidemic.[41] Neither Ramírez's report nor the accounts of the health commission make any reference to the mistaken judgment of his predecessor, nor do they blame the residents of Cazalla as having hidden information or misled the previous commissioner.

Instead, officials simply carried on with determining the extent of the new outbreak, working to contain it. All accounts and testimonies from Cazalla point to a broad and somewhat vague definition of what was or was not a dangerous illness. Doctor Salvador Esteban Nieto testified that there had been "contagious diseases" (*las enfermedades contagiosas*) in town since the previous month, pointing especially to "*landres* and *carbunclos* and *tavardete*, which are contagious illnesses." His colleague Doctor Hernando Vázquez testified to having treated "many with common illnesses and others with carbuncles and swellings indicating pestilential illness" (*muchas personas de unas enfermedades comunes y a otras de unos carbunclos y unas apostemas a maneras de el mal contagioso pestilencial*).[42]

While the previous commissioner to visit Cazalla de la Sierra had focused on whether or not the town was taking proper preventive measures such as burning all clothing and bedding belonging to those who had been sick, Ramírez paid more attention to treatment, visiting the town's pharmacists and questioning them about recent prescriptions filled, particularly those used for plague. Here again, he gained remarkably detailed information on how many prescriptions had been brought in, by whom they were brought, and for what illnesses. His report to the health commission showed the town suffering an outbreak of plague, which this time the people of Cazalla de la Sierra made no effort to conceal. And though several witnesses believed that the worst was over, it is important to note that none at this time attempted to gloss over their recent sufferings. In this light, the previous declarations of health by town leaders or doctors were not necessarily false efforts to manipulate the political relationship, but were a reflection of their genuine belief that no danger of plague existed. In addition, Seville's council had reports from two different investigators that confirmed the positive view in March.

Ramírez's report, again more than thirty pages in length, is the last reference to Cazalla de la Sierra to be found in the records from 1582. More than four months after first being declared infected, the town remained under suspicion and quarantine. Exactly when the health commission of Seville normalized its trade relations with Cazalla de la Sierra is unclear, one of many stories left unfinished by the documents. That the commission would have done so, however, is undoubted, for the changes in relations were never permanent. Like the plague commission itself, quarantines were temporary measures taken only when deemed necessary.

Despite the lack of closure for this particular story, it nonetheless helps to illuminate the effects that plague had on the political relations between Seville and the towns of its municipal territory. In their position of dominance, the councilmen of Seville controlled the terms of their coexistence. They held the power to determine the openness of relations and to impose municipal quarantines. This power was tempered, though, by the flexibility they were willing to use in adjusting those regulations.

Municipal quarantines, despite their harsh rhetoric, certainly did not cut off communication, and often only slowed down trade. At the same time, as we have seen in the previous chapter, a variety of individuals were able to circumvent the effects of these quarantines through direct petitions to the health commission.

Regional Negotiations

Local officials as well as residents in the towns and villages of Seville's tierra reacted with predictable unhappiness when denied their traditional trade rights, and were understandably frightened at the prospect of starvation if quarantined. But epidemics often stretched across greater spaces than the immediate tierra. In the years 1599 and 1600, plague could be found spread across the entire Iberian peninsula from the southern cities of Andalucía to the northern provinces of Galicia and Catalonia. There is evidence, in fact, that in these years a large portion of Western Europe experienced plague outbreaks of varying duration and severity.[43] In such times city leaders, in Seville as in all cities, had to be concerned with distant neighbors as well as those nearby. Communication and negotiation between local officials in nearly all towns and cities expanded in these years, as communities sought to balance their concerns about disease with their need to remain socially and economically integrated in the region. In both 1582 and 1600, Seville's plague commission negotiated not only with local officials from towns in their jurisdiction, but also with officials in many other cities and towns across the broader region of Andalucía, including Córdoba, Granada, Écija, Loja, Ronda, and Sanlúcar la Barrameda.

During these years of widespread plague, it became increasingly difficult for officials in most cities to maintain current and accurate information on which areas suffered plague and which did not. There were only so many health commissioners to be sent out, and as more and more rumors of plague in other cities circulated, so also communication between officials in various cities expanded. In such times, city officials often relied on rumor or news of an outbreak of plague in a distant city or town as sufficient reason to quarantine them, closing down trade and forbidding entry to their residents, at least until further investigations could be carried out.

By 1600, the clerk of the health commission no longer wrote out instructions for protecting the city from contagion, but printed them up in official handbills that could be distributed and posted. The instructions from that year encompassed five pages of orders that included a double-tiered system of gate guards and a mounted patrol of overseers, as well as directions on which gates and roads would be open, the times they would be open to traffic, and the manner of guarding them.[44] The instructions also included explicit directions on what the gate guards should do if they heard news or rumor of plague in a town or city that was not already declared infected and was not being guarded against. They were to immediately report this news to the lieutenant governor, who would investigate to verify or deny the rumor. In the meantime, any persons coming from the suspect area were to be denied entry until a decision was reached. In this way, Seville's health commissioners became involved in negotiations with officials in the city of Granada.

A resident of Granada, traveling to Seville in April of 1600, found himself detained at one of Seville's city gates, despite the fact that he carried official papers, which he believed to be sufficient identification. Unable to gain access to the city, and refusing to take no for an answer, he petitioned the health commission on April 10 for permission to enter the city.[45] The commission again chose to hear out the case, gather information, and then make an informed decision. It issued an order the following day for Alonso Leandro de Herrera to visit Granada and investigate. While this meant that the petitioner had to wait idly several days outside Seville until a verdict was reached, the commission was careful to limit Leandro and his assistants to just ten days to travel there, investigate, and report back.[46] Leandro had just returned from another trip, having visited five towns within the *tierra* to check on plague precautions, when he received his new orders. The day after turning in his account to the council for this previous trip so that he could be paid, he began his trip to Granada.[47]

As Leandro and his two assistants were traveling to Granada, however, city officials there were already working to renegotiate their relationship with Seville. Having heard of the ban on their citizens at Seville, Granada's officials acted quickly to address what they perceived to be unnecessary restrictions. Rather than wait for a representative from Seville, Granada's officials, much like those in Cazalla de la Sierra, took matters into their own hands. Over the course of four days, city officials gathered testimony from one councilman, eight physicians, one surgeon, four priests, four Jesuits, and four citizens of Seville who were at the time resident in Granada.[48] Each of these witnesses gave the same testimony. In the words of the cover letter that accompanied them, "this city has had and continues to have, by the grace of God, complete health, without a single case of contagion or even the suspicion thereof."[49] Officials sent these testimonies to Seville on April 18, two days after the arrival of Alonso Leandro de Herrera. However, as he himself wrote to the health commission, he began his inquiry by "secretly" visiting the different parishes of the city and asking the priests about recent deaths. This secret inquiry, which turned up no recent deaths or illnesses, was followed by formal interviews. Having learned of the lengthy testimonies already sent to the commission, Leandro chose to speak with only six local doctors, each of whom confirmed the health of the city.[50]

One of the doctors interviewed by Leandro admitted that some two months previously, a number of people in one of the poor outlying neighborhoods, known as San Lázaro, had suffered from typhus (*tabardete*) and what he referred to as malicious fevers (*calenturas malecciosas*), which he blamed on their poverty and lack of wholesome foods. He was careful to assert, however, that none of the cases could be considered plague (*peste*), as they did not exhibit the "necessary symptoms or conditions."[51] He went on to say that while fourteen or fifteen had died, nearly thirty recovered after being treated. Since that time, the residents of San Lázaro had remained entirely healthy for over twenty days, and the rest of Granada was even healthier. The other witnesses interviewed by Leandro chose, perhaps wisely, to focus only on the state of the city at that moment in time. No others referred to previous illnesses, and all asserted the complete health of Granada's residents. On April 24, four days after Alonso Leandro de Herrera had sent in his report, Seville's health commission voted to remove Granada from the list of infected cities.

In interviewing various officials in Granada, Leandro learned that the city counted itself healthy in part because of the care officials had been taking to restrict entrance to their city. One of the cities against which Granada guarded lay between Granada and Seville, the city of Loja. At least one official voiced his doubt on the need for Loja's quarantine, and Leandro decided to stop there on his way back to Seville in order to see for himself. Here again, a parallel course of events was playing out. Loja's administrators, knowing that their residents were being kept out of Granada, had already begun efforts to persuade Granada's officials of their health. They had compiled testimony from eleven residents: two doctors, one surgeon, two apothecaries, three barbers, and three priests, and sent copies to both Granada and Seville.[52]

Stopping on his return to Seville, Alonso Leandro de Herrera interviewed three men: the two doctors and one surgeon who had previously testified. The story told by the first witness, Dr. Alonso Sanchez, demonstrates the dilemma all municipal officials had to face. Testifying on April 22, Dr. Sanchez confirmed that during Lent of that year he had been called to treat a young boy who subsequently had died. Because the boy's grandmother, visiting from another town, had also recently died, the local officials of Loja reacted quickly. Fearing plague, they ordered the house to be shut up and the remaining family members removed to quarters outside of the city. According to Dr. Sanchez, this was all unnecessary and served only to spur rumors of plague in Loja. This news then spread quickly, putting Loja at risk of being quarantined by any number of other cities. Already Granada was preventing their residents from gaining entry, and they feared that soon Seville would do the same. In fact, Seville's council did initially list Loja as infected, but upon review a few days later councilmen removed Loja from their list.[53]

In the same year, 1600, the plague commission of Seville also recognized the widespread threat of plague and stretched its investigations more broadly than previously, including into Portugal. In January, the commission sent Diego Guillermo de Puebla to southern Portugal to investigate which towns there were infected and which maintained health. Portugal had come under control of the Spanish crown in 1580, during the reign of Philip II, following the death without heirs of the elderly King Henrique I. Commissioners, then, were not intruding on foreign officials, but investigating another local region. Puebla's report back to the commission at the end of the following month provided a listing of eighteen towns or cities known to be healthy (including Lisbon), and six suffering plague (*lugares apestados*), including Évora.[54]

Spring of 1600 brought illnesses across southern Spain and increased rumors of plague. At the same time that they investigated the situation in Granada and Loja, Seville's officials received testimonial collections from officials and doctors in Olvera and Ronda asserting the health of each.[55] Seville's councilmen also faced the opposite side of this issue, defending their own residents and residents of some towns within their jurisdiction as healthy and posing no risk of spreading plague to other places. When the city received news that the town of Marchena refused entry to residents of Utrera, which lay within Seville's jurisdiction, they agreed to write a testimonial letter on behalf of Utrera. This letter not only confirmed the health of the town, but specifically pointed out that soldiers (long seen as a danger to carry disease) sent there for quartering previously had not entered the city but remained outside.[56]

These examples demonstrate just some of the letters, petitions, and reports received and sent by Seville's health commission, and represent a small fraction of the communication flowing between the cities and towns of Andalucía. The politics of plague depended on reliable information and careful evaluation. There was no overall standard of health by which these cities evaluated one another, they depended on their own sources of information and their own measures of what constituted safety or danger. While the crown occasionally intervened in health matters, ordering for example that a certain city be considered healthy and removed from the list of those banned, most communication was directly between city councils that maintained autonomy in making quarantine decisions.[57] While such autonomy gave city governments the ability to tailor restrictions and negotiations according to local needs and concerns, it also increased the amount of time and effort each city had to put into defending itself when healthy. News of Granada's apparent outbreak, for example, had clearly spread across large areas, for in the statement of certification that accompanied the copies of the testimonies sent to Seville, the notary referred to the need for "two or more authentic copies . . . to be sent to Seville and other areas."[58] As there was no central body to coordinate information on health and illness, all cities relied on word of mouth to gain initial information on plague outbreaks, then later relied on firsthand reports from their own councilmen to confirm or deny the rumors. In this way, the threat of isolation that could seemingly result from plague restrictions in reality created a flood of letters, petitions, visits, and testimonies that crossed and overlapped as information flowed from city to city, and each municipality continually renegotiated its position.

These petitions demonstrate a complex economy and a highly mobile society that depended on long distance as well as local trade. The responses to them reflect an approach to plague and public health far more logical, careful, and flexible than often recognized. In guarding against plague, the commission was careful to gather as much information as possible before making their decisions. They preferred to err on the side of caution, thus they did often cut off trade with a nearby town or distant city simply on the basis of a rumor of plague. Yet at the same time, individual commissioners worked fairly tirelessly in traveling, interviewing, observing, and reporting so that the commission could be as well informed as possible. Most important, the commission remained entirely amenable to changing its opinion, altering its warnings, and removing towns and cities from the lists of those banned, once it had received what it felt was reliable information that the threat had passed.

The greatest difficulty for officials lay not in their lack of access to information, but rather lack of certainty in diagnosis. Repeatedly, doctors either disagreed on causes of illness or erred on the side of caution if it could be plague. The repercussions, however, could be quite difficult for other residents, as shown in the case of Loja. But the fear that still surrounded the possibility of plague meant that officials were obliged to take action or face the potential of a widespread epidemic they couldn't control. This meant a constant shuffling of bans and quarantines, sending officials across territories, their letters and testimonies constantly crossing back and forth. What is most striking is the tremendous effort officials put into protecting public health. In a sense, the system of quarantines and travel bans simply created more work for them, but it was work they willingly took on and carried out faithfully. Not until the late seventeenth century did the crown step in to centralize information on outbreaks and issue decrees on plague prevention measures.

Chapter Five

City and Crown

Balancing Authorities

In June 1581, King Philip II received a lengthy complaint about misman-agement of a public health crisis in Seville during an ongoing epidemic. This was the epidemic that later chroniclers attributed to catarrh (*catarro*), which spread virulently beginning in 1580 and was still prevalent the next year.[1] This complaint, however, talks not only of a vague contagion, but specifically refers to plague (*mal de peste*) and the dangers of its spread. The complaint began by acknowledging the good intentions of the royally appointed *Asistente*, but castigated all other municipal officials as neglectful. In particular, it specifically charged the *Alguacil mayor* (public safety official) and his assistant with neglect and absenteeism that had enabled a recent crime wave, including thieves breaking into houses and an unusual number of deaths (the causes of which were not specified). The city councilmen, both *Veintiquatros* and *Jurados*, stood accused of neglecting their duties as well, leaving residents to suffer the "downfall and ruin" of the city (*ruyna y perdicion de este lugar*), including a lack of sanitation that had led to dan-gerous levels of filth clogging the streets. Continuing the list of complaints, the letter asserted an overall neglect of the city that meant houses were not properly closed after a diagnosis of plague, the sick who had been removed outside city walls were allowed back in too easily, and families were illegally unloading bedding or clothing from the sick by dumping them in the pla-zas by night, to be taken by poor beggars unaware they could die from the disease transmitted by these items.[2] While in many ways the tone of the com-plaint sounds exaggerated today, it raised what were likely some valid points. Just as important as the specific issues raised is the method used to chal-lenge official laxity, by drawing royal attention to municipal governance. For much of the early modern era, Spanish rulers maintained a watchful aware-ness of plague outbreaks, in particular any that occurred close to Madrid.[3] But by and large, they made no effort to dictate public health policy to city officials. Epidemics remained a local issue to be managed on a daily basis by those with firsthand knowledge of the area, and the crown intervened only when directly asked to do so. In response to this complaint, the king's secretary, Matteo Vazquez, sent a copy (without revealing the original author) to city officials along with a request for explanation.[4] After some discussion, officials compiled their response, defending their actions and efforts. This satisfied the king, who conveyed his contentment with all that city officials had done to combat the epidemic, and who made no effort to interfere further in municipal oversight of the epidemic.[5]

Throughout the early modern era, public health, particularly the management of epidemics, remained first and foremost a municipal concern. Although royal interest in protecting the health of the public became evident in the late medieval era, as rulers in both Aragon and Castile adopted educational and licensing controls for medical practitioners, the task of setting policies, administering public hospitals, and deciding how best to prevent the spread of disease within the cities rested with municipal authorities.[6] From the fourteenth to the seventeenth centuries, the crown's role in epidemic management was minimal, generally limited to occasional advice from court physicians. The lack of effort by early modern rulers to establish a centralized policy for epidemic response is, at least in part, another reflection of the complexity of disease beliefs in the early modern era. Epidemics arose in response to local conditions, a complex and often chaotic combination of sin, stench, climate, and individual temperament. Prevention and treatment for these epidemics needed the constant attention of local officials to implement, monitor, and adjust them according to continually changing circumstances.

Beginning in the last half of the sixteenth century, though, both the crown and city officials began to grant a greater role to the crown in directing epidemics. This series of incremental changes increased the crown's role in both monitoring outbreaks of plague and helping determine quarantine policies, areas once reserved exclusively for municipal authorities. Based on an older tradition of regulating medical practice (education and licensing), the crown broadened its role to regulating other aspects of public health. By the end of the sixteenth century, near the end of Philip II's reign, the crown increasingly offered advice to city leaders, and at the same time these municipal authorities increasingly turned to the crown to intervene in disputes between cities over quarantine policies. This trend continued in the seventeenth century, under Philip III (r. 1598–1621) and Philip IV (r. 1621–65), then escalated after midcentury, during the reign of Charles II (r. 1665–1700), as the crown began to issue standard printed orders to municipal officials declaring which cities and towns were considered infected, and what measures officials should take to protect their territories. The beginnings of this shift may be attributed to Philip II's efforts to take direct control of as many issues as possible, and his personal correspondence with officials in Seville shows this hands-on approach. But the continued and increased intervention of the crown in local issues of public health seems likely the result of an opposite movement away from personal rule. In contrast to Philip II's intensely personal rule, subsequent Hapsburg rulers of the seventeenth century are all known for delegating decision-making powers first to their court favorites, and subsequently through those favorites to governing councils.[7] Thus it seems likely that the motivation for the increased intervention of the crown in epidemic issues came not from the kings themselves, but from those surrounding them at court, perhaps from court physicians or other advisors.

This increased role of the crown in epidemics likely also reflects a changed view of the state that emerged in this same era. In France, the shift to centralized control began in the mid-seventeenth century with regional authorities, the *parlements* and *intendants*, then moved further inward to the crown's inner circle, overseen by Jean-Baptiste Colbert.[8] In midcentury Spain, a similar centralization of policy formed under the Council of Castile, which increasingly took on the role of coordinating information on epidemics, issuing standard orders and monitoring internal trade relations in times of plague. The arrival of (what would later be determined as) the last significant plague outbreak in Western Europe, that of Marseille in 1720, encouraged the new Bourbon king, Philip V (r. 1700–1746), to approve the creation of the *Junta Suprema de Sanidad* to oversee and coordinate epidemic prevention throughout the peninsula. The Bourbon dynasty, which had taken control in Spain following the War of Spanish Succession (1700–1712), is known for reforming many aspects of administration not only in Madrid, but also in the colonial territories of the Americas. It would therefore be easy to see this shift from municipal control of epidemics to crown control as merely one more Bourbon reform. In reality, however, the shift toward crown intervention began in the late sixteenth century, as rulers gradually took a greater interest in overseeing plague regulation.

Crown Regulation of Medicine

The Spanish crown(s) had long asserted royal prerogative in some issues of medical education and licensing. Although the advent of direct crown control over medical licensing is generally dated to the creation in 1477 of a governing board, the *Tribunal de Protomedicato*, there is plentiful evidence of earlier assertions of royal rights of control. Among these is the 1225 *Fuero Real* of Castile, which in essence delegated this royal control to municipal officials.[9] But medieval efforts to assert royal control over medical practice are generally seen as ineffective or merely sporadic, in part because until the fifteenth century the Iberian Peninsula remained fractured into several kingdoms.[10] The 1469 marriage of Fernando and Isabel united the future rulers

of Aragon and Castile, and with their ascensions to their respective thrones
in 1474 and 1479, these corulers affirmed their claim over the majority of
the Iberian Peninsula. Building on a foundation laid by Juan II of Castile
(r. 1406–54), Fernando and Isabel established the *Protomedicato* in Castile
specifically to extend royal control over medical licensing for a wide variety
of practitioners, including physicians, surgeons, apothecaries, spice dealers,
and bonesetters. In so doing, they reasserted the crown's right to control
the educational requirements of medical practitioners, to determine who
did or did not have the right to practice, and to decide complaints against
practitioners.[11] Composed initially of four examiners, known first as *alcaldes
examinadores* and later as *protomédicos*, the board worked to establish licensing
standards across the medical marketplace in Castile. While municipal officials did not acquiesce lightly to sharing or losing the power to license, the
crown persisted in its efforts at centralization.[12]

Subsequent Spanish monarchs of the sixteenth and seventeenth centuries continued to reshape both medical education and licensing control
through the *Protomedicato*. In 1523, Charles V placed the first limits on the
protomédicos of Castile, reducing the territory over which they held rights to
examine to the court and five leagues surrounding. But for the next thirty
years, this restriction was not as limiting as it may sound, for the Spanish
crown had no established capital until 1561, and instead periodically stayed
in various cities. Therefore, the *protomédicos* continued to have jurisdiction
over a fairly extensive, albeit shifting, territory. In any case, petitioners continued to travel from distant areas to the court specifically to request an
examination and license from the *Protomedicato*, perhaps either in a bid to
overcome local restrictions or to provide them with mobility to practice in
any city.[13] The 1523 regulations also limited the kinds of practitioners who
fell under regulation by the *Protomedicato* to physicians, surgeons, apothecaries, and barbers, specifically leaving out midwives, spice dealers, bonesetters,
and faith healers.[14] At the same time, however, Charles oversaw the expansion of medical regulation with new appointments of *protomédicos* in Spanish
Italian territories including Milan, Savoy, Parma, Naples, and Sicily. Within
Spain, Charles made separate appointments in Navarre and Valencia in an
attempt (not necessarily successful) to likewise maintain crown control in
those regions.[15]

Philip II took a more active interest in health matters, continually asserting
his royal authority through a wide range of issues relating to medical education, licensing, and practice.[16] During his reign the *Protomedicato* expanded
its power to more effectively adjudicate complaints, prosecute misconduct,
and enforce medical legislation. In addition, Philip II expanded control
over both university training and nonacademic empiricism, establishing
both new curricula standards for medical schools and new ways that practitioners without formal training could prove the efficacy of empiric cures.[17]

Yet while the Spanish Hapsburg rulers retained a strong interest in aspects of medical practice, particularly education and licensing, the bulk of administrative power for health issues remained with local municipal officials.

Those municipal leaders complained frequently and vociferously to the crown about problems with the system of licensing under the *Protomedicato*, generally when they felt their control over local affairs threatened by royal interference.[18] As shown in chapter 1, Seville's officials, like those in most other cities, involved themselves directly in health care, taking control of hiring doctors, nurses, and pharmacists to tend to the poor and incarcerated. In addition, the city council monitored pharmacies by routinely commissioning councilmen to accompany local physicians to inspect the pharmacies, checking the remedies on hand for freshness and efficacy.[19] The council also sought to maintain standards of health care by hearing complaints about misconduct or mismanagement. In 1584, for example, the council members heard a complaint from a Dr. Estrada, a new arrival in Seville from Madrid, about the teaching of surgeon Bartolomé Hidalgo de Agüero, whose methods Estrada deemed dangerous.[20] In this case, the complaint was not upheld, and Hidalgo de Agüero went on to write a well-known treatise on surgery, credited today as innovative for its time. The intervention of the city council in all these health matters demonstrates the important role of local, rather than royal, officials in matters relating to medical practice. Local officials also held firm control over monitoring and responding to local epidemics.

Epidemics

Just as Philip II played a more active role in medical education and licensing, he likewise established a precedent for more active crown intervention in epidemics.[21] Certainly, Philip II maintained far more frequent correspondence with royally appointed governors, or other municipal officials, than had his predecessors, particularly during times of plague.[22] Employing more physicians and surgeons at court than had previous rulers, Philip II relied on them not only for their knowledge and skills at court, but also to offer that same knowledge and experience more widely through written treatises.[23] In 1582, court physicians Francisco Valles and Antonio Fernández de Vitoria offered a brief memorial on avoiding the spread of plague to Seville's city council; Philip II sent another memorial from Valles to Barcelona's council in 1589.[24] Such memorials were purely advisory, of course, and did not carry the weight of royal decrees. Yet they mark an important step in the crown's growing role in public health, an effort to establish a standard understanding of and response to epidemics.

By the turn of the century, the outbreak known as the Atlantic plague (roughly 1596–1603), prompted widespread interest in plague prevention and treatment. Appearing first in northern Europe, this epidemic spread in several directions, eventually infecting most of France, England, and Spain. The outbreak spared the areas encircling the Mediterranean, spreading instead along the Atlantic coasts, moving inland at a rapid pace.[25] In Spain, plague jumped southward along sea routes, arriving in Santander in 1596, emerging the next year in numerous coastal cities from Bilbao to Lisbon, soon followed by the Atlantic ports of Andalucía, including Cádiz and Seville. From 1598 onward, the northern and central inland Spanish regions including Galicia, Asturias, Extremadura, and Castile likewise suffered. The widespread nature of this outbreak, occurring at the end of Philip II's reign and continuing during that of Philip III, may well have further influenced the crown to expand its role in coordinating information from one area of Spain to another.

As plague spread across these vast territories, cities from Oviedo to Seville reacted as they had for centuries, each implementing its own program of plague restrictions meant to protect healthy residents and limit contact with the sick.[26] In many ways, this is one of the easiest epidemics to study, as city officials generated reams of paperwork related to it, recording events within the cities, keeping track of municipal expenditures, and maintaining correspondence with the crown.[27] Both Philip II and (after September 1598) Philip III maintained close correspondence with civic and medical leaders in cities surrounding Madrid, requesting frequent updates on their health.[28] Officials in cities such as Burgos, Ávila, Valladolid, Segovia, and Toledo offered the crown continual updates on the state of health in their cities as well as information on how they were responding to the crisis.[29] In addition, both rulers again encouraged court physicians and surgeons to publish new treatises related to plague. Surgeon Antonio Pérez published a small treatise in 1598, the same year that Philip II requested a similar treatise from his principle physician, Luis Mercado. Mercado initially wrote in Latin for learned physicians, but quickly produced a translation in Castilian for publication the next year, in order to make it accessible to a wider audience.[30] Cristóbal Pérez de Herrera's 1599 treatise, *Dubitationes ad maligni, popularisque morbi*, raised questions on the best methods of treatment for plague, which led to a brief dispute at court. The crown again intervened, calling together eleven court physicians and surgeons, Drs. Zamudio de Alfaro, Porras, Bermejo, Orozco, Salinas, Espinosa, Pérez, Montemayor, Sepúlveda, Sosa, and Herrera, to debate these issues. The result was a short treatise by Andrés Zamudio de Alfaro, also published in 1599.[31]

Court practitioners were not the only ones offering their opinions on this epidemic. The Atlantic plague prompted a flood of plague treatises all across Spain. In his study of plague and physicians in Spain between 1475 and 1610, Antonio Carreras Panchón notes thirty-nine treatises published on plague between 1597 and 1603. In Seville, at least eleven medical writers published works on plague in those same years, and treatises published nearby, such as those of Alonso de Freilas in Jaén and Miguel Franco in Córdoba, would likely have circulated in Seville as well. The authors of these treatises varied, from the apothecary and distiller Diego Santiago to the chairs of medicine at the university, Juan de Carvajal and Juan Saavedra. The remainder were practicing physicians, each of whom offered their own explanations of causes and treatments for plague based in their experiences.[32]

There was little advice the royal physicians could offer municipal officials that was new or different from what they already carried out. Quarantines, limiting travelers and goods from areas declared infected, and other similar measures had, as we have seen, a long history throughout Europe. What does seem to change after the Atlantic plague was a greater interest by the crown of the extent of such outbreaks, and a greater role in reestablishing forms of normalcy when plague had subsided. Thus, in the early seventeenth century, the crown did not direct the imposition of municipal quarantines, but it did begin to regulate the lifting of such quarantines in response to appeals from affected cities. The movement from municipal to royal control of epidemics was gradual, culminating in the last quarter of the century.

Here again, Seville presents an interesting case study for examining the interplay of royal and municipal control of public health. Royal interests were well represented in Seville, as the crown appointed not only the head of the city council (*Asistente*), but also the authorities at the Casa de la Contratación, including the president, treasurer, purveyor, and lawyers.[33] It was the Casa that held the greatest importance and interest for the crown, as the body overseeing navigation, exploration, and trade with the New World. Officials at the Casa maintained a frequent and detailed correspondence with the crown, which kept the crown appraised of many events (including epidemics) within the city, although it focused principally on the provisioning and departure of the Indies fleets.[34] These fleets, scheduled to leave the city twice a year, could be delayed for a variety of reasons, which then needed to be explained to the king. Despite the detailed knowledge the crown received about epidemics in Seville, neither Philip II nor Philip III made any effort to intervene in how the city managed its affairs, even when the existence of epidemics threatened to delay the fleet's departure. In April 1581, for example, the president of the Casa notified Philip II that because of the epidemic then raging in the city, it was increasingly difficult to procure supplies for the outbound fleet, in part because so many had fled the city and in part because those who remained were little inclined to negotiate terms.[35] The court, in turn, repeatedly warned officials at the Casa to be careful not to allow the fleets to become contaminated by either persons or clothing that could propagate plague and carry it to the New World.[36] In the same month, when the president and officials at the Casa petitioned the king to be allowed to leave the city as so many others had already done, they were denied. They asked to relocate temporarily to the nearby town of Coria, which lay approximately two leagues south of Seville along the Guadalquivir River. Although they carefully argued that it offered not only a healthier environment, but also immediate access to all the ships coming or going, enabling them to continue working, they did not succeed in persuading Philip II, who ordered them to remain.[37]

These same royal officials often had a turbulent relationship with city officials, as they frequently found themselves in competition for resources, particularly in times of scarcity. Municipal quarantines affecting the flow of goods into the city were just one factor contributing to scarcity of food in the early modern era. The region of Andalucía also suffered periodic droughts and locust infestations that could seriously damage the wheat and barley crops, creating severe shortages that forced city officials to import grain from other areas. As previously discussed, grain shipped by sea often fell under suspicion as prone to corruption, so officials worked hard to acquire what they could from neighboring territories that could be carted overland by mules instead. But this often put them in competition with the royal officials at the Casa, who had the advantage of royal backing in commandeering whatever resources were available. In 1580, as the city suffered a grain shortage, Seville's officials had to petition the king to allow them to keep the wheat and barley they had already bought so that the Casa officials would not override them and requisition the grain for a fleet in Málaga.[38] Yet at other times, city councilmen found themselves battling against one of the Casa's principal officials, Francisco Duarte. In May 1581, Duarte seized carts of wheat bound for Seville, which had been stopped in the town of Constantina because of existing quarantine regulations. Although the wheat came from an uninfected area near Segovia, and therefore would have been allowed to continue its journey, Seville's officials had little choice but to look elsewhere to replace it.[39] The next month, Duarte appeared at a city council meeting, offering to sell the city surplus wheat that had been commandeered by the king to feed the army he had amassed to help fight for his claim to the Portuguese throne. When Philip succeeded in gaining the throne, he no longer need the supplies and authorized Duarte to make a sale to city officials.[40] Three months later, still embroiled in a dispute with city officials over whether the terms of that sale contract had been properly met, Duarte embargoed more grain that Seville had purchased, leaving city officials bereft and looking to import grain from Sicily or possibly North Africa.[41]

Direct Crown Intervention

By the late sixteenth century, the crown began to take a more active role in regulating relations between cities. There were two ways this shift began to occur. First was in the *Audiencias*, the royal appeals courts, which became a center for settling various disputes between towns or cities related to epidemics.[42] The second was that officials in towns and cities began to appeal directly to the crown for support in various ways. For example, in 1581, residents in Málaga appealed to the crown for permission to prohibit ships from Seville and Cádiz (areas known to be suffering epidemics) from entering Málaga's port for resupply.[43] On the other side of such disputes, city officials increasingly turned to the crown for assistance in reopening communication or trade. At the same time that residents in Málaga sought to protect themselves from potentially infected ships, officials in Seville sought crown support for their ability to trade. The areas surrounding Seville had imposed bans on Seville's residents, making it impossible to negotiate the purchase of wheat anywhere. In desperation, the city's *Asistente*, the Conde de Villar, appealed to the king to order towns of Andalucía to resume trading grain with the city's representatives.[44] Both these cases reflect a view of the crown as a sort of last resort when normal channels of negotiation did not provide a satisfactory outcome for one side or the other. Thus, the crown began to assume a larger role during epidemics not by imposing or enforcing regulations directly on the cities, but rather as arbiter of disputes over the ability of local officials to enforce their regulations. While the exact parameters of this expanding role remain to be studied, there is tantalizing evidence of other cities across Castile likewise turning to royal authority.[45]

Just after the turn of the century, as the Atlantic plague slowly tapered out and normal routines returned, the crown played an increased role in helping cities reestablish trade networks. In April 1600, officials in Ronda compiled testimony from four local doctors and one surgeon asserting the complete return to health of their city, successfully using these to petition the crown for a royal cedula confirming their right to resume trade with other cities and towns. In May 1600, authorities in the city of Lisbon successfully petitioned the *Audiencia* to have their town removed from Seville's list of infected areas.[46] Three years later, in January 1603, the crown responded to an appeal by officials in Córdoba, issuing a royal directive declaring Córdoba healthy, and ordering cities and towns to allow free entry to its residents and goods.[47] There is no evidence that the crown in any of these cases relied on any more information than what these municipal officials provided themselves, yet the crown nonetheless showed a new willingness to step in to arbitrate such disputes.

By 1630, the crown faced a new threat, the possibility of conspiracies to deliberately spread plague. The belief that some people had knowledge of how to manufacture powders or salves that could deliberately spread plague dated back to the emergence of plague in the fourteenth century. Such beliefs in the fourteenth century led leaders in many European communities to persecute Jews, accusing them of poisoning wells. Although sometimes considered a part of witchcraft, accusations of spreading plague were, in fact, a separate category of accusations and continued sporadically through the fifteenth and sixteenth centuries in various parts of Europe.[48]

It was in response to such fears and accusations that the Spanish crown made an early effort to issue centralized control measures aimed at preventing foreigners from bringing this "pestis manufacta" into Spain. In June 1630, officials in Milan, after receiving reports of suspicious behavior, arrested a man on charges of spreading poisonous plague powders. Upon interrogation and torture, the man implicated another as an accomplice and the two were found guilty and executed.[49] By September, Philip IV began issuing decrees denouncing the "enemies of the human race" who would propagate such poisons and offering rewards to anyone who could name the guilty parties, as well as immunity to anyone who immediately confessed to being an accomplice.[50] In an October decree to leaders in several cities, including Seville and Córdoba, the king offered a double incentive of both rewards to those who would come forth with information, accompanied with the threat of loss of goods or even one's life for not sharing information with authorities.[51] Citing the recent influx of foreigners who had stressed municipal resources, the king also ordered all foreigners who had arrived since August 1 to declare themselves to officials, who would then decide whether they had legitimate cause to remain.

Although these fears were, of course, for naught, and indeed no epidemic resulted in Spain in 1630, these events reflect both the ongoing fear of plague through the seventeenth century and the increasing role of the crown in keeping municipal leaders informed of events. By the 1670s, the Spanish crown had begun to centralize epidemic response by collecting and distributing information about existing outbreaks and issuing orders for a standard set of preventive measures.[52] There was nothing particularly innovative in these royal orders, they continued to reflect traditional standards of travel ban and quarantine. What changed was the effort by the crown to act as central clearinghouse of information, sharing news of plague outbreaks in more distant cities. These royal decrees, ordering the cessation of trade with certain cities, still relied, however, on local authorities to use the information and implement preventive measures.

This shift from municipal control to crown control of epidemics is mirrored in both England and France. The earliest attempt at centralized control over plague measures seems to have emerged in England. Ironically, though, Paul Slack, the historian who has documented the impact of plague there, argued for England's "backwardness" in responding to plague. He states that "England was unlike many other European countries in having no public precautions against plague at all before 1518. By comparison with Italy or France, it was in this respect a benighted, backward country, as anxious foreign visitors often remarked."[53] If, indeed, local leaders in English towns and cities made no effort to create a system of plague response, then

England may be seen as lagging behind. But in examining the creation of *centralized* plague regulation established or authorized by the crown, which is what Slack actually describes, England stands out as an early exemplar. Although these first efforts in 1518 were not terribly effective, later and more successful efforts in 1578 and 1603 still put the English crown at the forefront of European monarchies in this respect.

In France, regulation of epidemics remained under municipal control until the 1620s, when the parlements, especially in Paris, began to issue directives. Yet while the parlements may been seen as reflective of greater centralized power, they remained regional authorities rather than national ones. At midcentury the French crown begin to assert authority over epidemic control, which scholars have tied to the rise of French mercantilism, as evidenced by the involvement of the French minister Jean-Baptiste Colbert in coordinating plague response from the 1660s onward.[54]

Definitive change in Spain came in the eighteenth century, after the rise of the Bourbon dynasty to the throne. Philip V, the first Bourbon ruler, oversaw the creation of the Junta Suprema de Sanidad in 1720, specifically in response to the outbreak of plague in Marseilles.[55] Trade ships from the Levant brought plague once more to the Mediterranean, creating a new outbreak in the spring of 1720. By this time, authorities across Europe had all become much more attuned to the dangers of widespread epidemics, and began watching carefully the unfolding epidemic in southern France. As French authorities created a cordon sanitaire around the city, effectively forbidding exit to residents, outside of France authorities likewise began to take precautions. In England, concern over this epidemic prompted the renewal of naval quarantine acts, despite sometimes fierce opposition.[56] Spain, given its closer proximity by both land and sea, faced greater concern. The Junta quickly set to work coordinating the protection of Spain's ports and borders from the contagion, creating a veritable flood of memoranda and instructions.[57] Whether a result of these measures or other factors, the epidemic was indeed contained to Marseille, though at a high cost to residents there.[58] While no further outbreaks of plague are recorded for Western Europe, plague remained longer in other areas, particularly parts of North Africa and the countries of the Levant. The Junta, therefore, continued diligent work monitoring outbreaks in these regions through the rest of the eighteenth century.[59] As the threat of plague gradually faded, however, many other public health threats emerged, especially yellow fever, which occupied the Junta for the remainder of the century.[60]

Conclusion

The plagues and pestilence of the early modern era continue to fascinate in part because they defy clear definition. Plague was more than a diagnosis, it was a multifaceted and changeable idea that held many different, and sometimes conflicting, meanings. Both feared and ignored, it was a constant, albeit not a continual, threat. Perceived as both unpredictable and yet controllable, its effects were felt in nearly all aspects of European life for several centuries. This particular complexity of plague, taken within a more generally complex understanding of all disease, gave rise to an intricate system of public health that depended on cooperative effort by both authorities and residents.

The disruptive and often devastating effects of plague have been well-documented. The intense fear, isolation, and abandonment vividly described by fourteenth-century chroniclers, picked up and recounted by historians in later centuries, continues to shape a common understanding of the Black Death and the subsequent plague era. This study seeks not to erase those negative images, but merely to add another perspective to them—that of acceptance and adaptation. In a way that no other disease did, plague forced early modern populations to adapt their routines, attitudes, and expectations to its persistent threat.

The study of plague has been traditionally framed by two distinct but intertwined contexts, that of a communal crisis and that of a medical crisis. As a communal crisis, the fear of epidemics created chaos by encouraging self-preservation, breaking down social bonds (the abandonment often chronicled from the Black Death), and placing sufficient stress on cultural and religious traditions that many of these traditions changed or gradually disappeared. These studies emphasize the tragedy of loss, relying on chronicles and personal accounts to reconstruct the horror and fear created by plague. In this traditional view, plague became the bridge between the medieval and Renaissance eras, erasing old traditions and mentalities, giving room for the new attitudes or beliefs of the Renaissance.[1] At the very least, the Black Death has often been used as a marking point between the late medieval and early modern eras.[2]

As a medical crisis, plague has been credited with provoking a turn to modernity, giving rise to public health systems that directly addressed disease and its potential to spread. Civic authorities, backed up by medical men, encouraged the growth of a nascent modern medical bureaucracy to oversee issues of public health far beyond the traditional ones of sanitation and the regulation of food, water, and medicines. What had once been a private matter (health and disease) now became a public concern. While previous diseases, notably leprosy, had aroused public concerns about possible transmission of disease from the sick to the healthy, plague reinforced the trend because it represented a much stronger threat to the community at large. Leprosy festered, infecting relatively fewer numbers, then disfigured and disabled victims before slowly killing them; plague spread widely and rapidly, then quickly decimated those infected. Thus while efforts to protect public health started in the Middle Ages with the building of leprosaria to keep the infected at arm's length, the real impetus for state control came from plague. This new focus on communal health gave rise to the boards of health of the Italian city-states that worked to provide a consistent response to epidemics.

The rise of this state system of public health, however, also gave rise to new conflicts between individual and communal interests. So within the broader historiographical tradition of medical crisis has also come the framework of conflict in which authorities tried to impose regulations or restrictions while residents worked equally hard to thwart them. In this context, the selfishness and ignorance of individuals led them into frequent conflict with health authorities, which in turn could be seen as further endangering the community at large.[3]

In many ways, of course, both of these traditional interpretations are correct. Even as the chaos of the fourteenth-century Black Death gave way to more organized responses to epidemics in later centuries, epidemics often continued to provoke some amount of disorder, fear, and suspicion. Records of this, in all countries and languages, remain plentiful. Historians researching later epidemics from the fifteenth through the seventeenth centuries have pointed to records of social and economic disruption, even as both civic and medical authorities worked to impose order during epidemics. The two most famous late epidemics in London (1665) and Marseilles (1720) are both known for creating just such upheavals and increasing social splintering.[4]

This dual crisis framework, however, pays scant attention to the means by which Europeans learned to live with plague. Despite all best efforts, epidemics with varying mortality rates (whether defined as "pestilential" or not) continued to be a fact of life, one that the vast majority of the population had to learn to live through. Plague did not arrive and depart with any predictability or with any decisiveness. Rather, it was a sort of creeping fog that settled among populations, often rising and disappearing only to reappear at unpredictable moments. It was elusive, showing clearer signs to some than to others, and certainly more feared by some than others. While many noble or wealthy families could and did continue to remove themselves from cities during the worst epidemics, most people had no such choice. Instead, they adapted to the constant threat of disease.

In areas without permanent health boards, adaptation meant the development of a reconfigured system of public health that had to balance competing interests. In Seville, the temporary health commissions worked on both a materialist and symbolic level to monitor and prevent the spread of plague. A thriving early modern community depended on more than merely the health of the residents. It also required the maintenance of routines of communication, travel and exchange, and the ability of people to access work, markets, and family. These communities needed to be assured that officials were paying attention to outbreaks of "suspicious" disease and were working to provide protections against them. At the same time, individuals needed reassurance that their lives would not be brought to a standstill, that business and trade could continue, and that no undue penalty would be exacted from the healthy. Officials in Seville worked to accommodate the needs of both. Seville's city council, embracing the standard idea of separation of sick and healthy, maintained a routine of response to epidemics that depended on first enacting restriction, then reassessing whether such restrictions were still necessary in both individual and communal cases. This meant a continual process of collecting and evaluating information.

The public health response detailed in this book was one of practical action that demanded continual work by the city's officials. They responded to fears of pestilence by controlling what they could. They ordered and supervised the cleaning of the city, monitored illnesses, closed gates, and demanded papers from travelers. Above all, they investigated, reported, conferred, and acted. They attempted to protect the community by isolating or removing the sick individuals who could threaten the overall health of the group, when they felt it was necessary. The question of this necessity was one of the most difficult for them to determine, and their debates and delays in taking these actions reflect the challenges they faced in determining when plague was actually becoming epidemic and when there were mere "ordinary" illnesses with signs of pestilence. When officials did become convinced of a sufficient threat of an epidemic, they enacted restrictions. When those restrictions proved problematic, they investigated and cautiously reconsidered. They collected as much information as possible, and weighed the costs of their decisions. The records from the health commissioners reflect little fear of danger to themselves, and while the movements of strangers or foreigners (those from outside Seville) roused suspicion and investigation, they gave such travelers ample opportunities to plead their cases. Above all, officials in Seville demonstrated a surprising willingness to work with residents rather than merely dictating terms to them.

Beginning with closing city gates to monitor and limit traffic into the city, the council also watched surrounding communities carefully. Restrictions on travel were a means to maintain a greater sense of control and to give public demonstration of that control to the residents. But the restrictions were also flexible. That people affected by the imposition of plague restrictions would object to them and seek to evade them is not surprising. That large numbers would do so via official channels of petition, which required some time and patience, is more surprising. And that the city's health commissioners would listen to all complaints and petitions, regardless of how small, carefully investigate the circumstances of each, and be willing to work with residents is very surprising. But the system created by Seville's health officials seems to have worked quite well. Those who worked within it, seeking official waivers for the movement of both people and their goods, were successful, while those who attempted to move outside official scrutiny became subject to further investigation, often resulting in incarceration and fines. The large number of individual petitions that fill the records is a testimony to how willing residents were to utilize this system and work with officials rather than against them.

The most prominent group of those clearly willing to play by the rules were merchants, who had the greatest financial motive and stood to lose the most because of travel restrictions. They stand out in the records of petitions, working within official parameters to gain permission to move in and out of the city for both themselves and their goods. They voluntarily quarantined their goods outside the city, sought the appropriate paperwork for themselves, and worked within the restrictions to leverage their position. At the same time, it is striking that they didn't simply send their goods via carters, but themselves traveled in and out of areas with little concern for possible exposure to plague. In fact, travelers of all sorts, from both nearby towns and distant cities, continued to move about the countryside seemingly unconcerned by reports of plague. While municipal officials continued to be concerned about who might bring plague with them, many individuals showed little such concern for their own exposure to pestilence. Both merchant and naval ships continued to arrive in Seville, even at the height of epidemics, adapting their routines to accommodate whatever restrictions officials decided to impose. City officials themselves moved about both within the city and the surrounding countryside, even when plague had clearly been declared in those areas. Likewise, although stories of doctors and priests refusing to visit the sick are plentiful, the records in Seville also show members of both groups ready and willing to carry out those duties; monastic houses in Seville even appealed for permission to open city gates in order to gain access to the poorest neighborhoods outside the city walls, and confessed to climbing over the walls when necessary. It is, of course, impossible to generalize for all cases, but a strong argument can be made that such disregard for the dangers of plague was neither simple stupidity nor selfishness, but rather a reflection of the multifaceted understanding of "pestilence" and how it spread.

It is in looking carefully at the understanding of pestilence that the modern scholar sees most clearly the differences between early modern and modern understanding of disease. The presumed foundations of modernity often become shakiest here, as understanding plague in early modern terms is sometimes challenging. It was at once individual and communal, environmental and contagious, routine and deadly, a result of dietary deficiency and a result of bad weather. While many officials put great emphasis on the links of poverty to plague, physicians and surgeons continually debated the true nature of the disease.

In published treatises and in consultations with city officials, medical men in Seville offered a variety of views on the causes, symptoms, and best regimens for prevention and treatment, all of which show both the vagaries of diagnosis in this era and the intellectual liveliness of Seville's medical community. Though not directly in charge of public health in the city, Seville's physicians, surgeons, and apothecaries maintained a strong and visible role during epidemics. Acting as agents, consultants, and investigators, the city's doctors played a significant role in enabling much of the public health balance described in this book to continue. In their varying diagnoses, interpretations, and the range of causative factors to which they pointed, they continually recast a broad understanding of plague that allowed both officials and residents to adapt their routines of interaction.

This adaptation can be seen as a continual set of balances or tradeoffs, enacted by both officials and residents, though most would have been largely unaware they were doing so. For city officials, managing the city during epidemics meant collecting and balancing different forms of information: the expert opinions of physicians, the reports and requests of residents, the observations and reports of the councilmen who were out in the community, and the instructions of royal officials. For physicians, medical practice was a balance of interpretation between the theory they learned from Hippocratic and Galenic texts, the theory or advice they read in works of their contemporaries, and their own experiences with patients. For ordinary people, living in the plague era meant balancing their fears of disease with their need to continue to leave their houses and move about the city and countryside, even with pestilence in their midst. All of these issues of balance emerged simultaneously, interacted, and resulted in temporary social and economic shifts that enabled most routines of city life to continue. Above all, these efforts to find balance depended on the cooperative efforts of officials, physicians, and residents, and their willingness to open and maintain a variety of channels of communication.

Eventually the threat that plague posed would recede for another period of months, or if they were lucky, years. But the cycle of quarantine and negotiation would continue to shape municipal life both within the city and across the broader region. Those negotiations, and the continued ability of individuals and communities to pursue them, depended directly on shared perceptions of what public health meant in the sixteenth century and the best means of providing for it.

Notes

Introduction

1. The Centers for Disease Control publishes a leading journal in this field, *Emerging Infectious Diseases*, http://www.cdc.gov/ncidod/eid/index.htm. See also Garrett, *The Coming Plague*; Drexler, *Emerging Epidemics*; Quammen, *Spillover*; Jones et al., "Global Trends in Emerging Infectious Diseases."

2. Many such cases have occurred in the last decade, a sample of news stories would include: De Lollis and Kessler, "False Alarm"; Centers for Disease Control and Prevention "Update: Severe Acute Respiratory Syndrome"; Bluestein, "Man in 2007 TB Scare"; "Avian Flu Timeline."

3. See Baldwin, *Contagion and the State*.

4. Despite a history of some dispute, these epidemics have long been identified as caused by bubonic plague. This view has in recent years been bolstered by new microbiological studies (see note 9 below). Plague is traditionally viewed as affecting Europe in three major pandemics. The first was in the ancient world, recurring in cycles from the so-called Plague of Justinian (541–42) to the mid-eighth century. See Little, *Plague and the End of Antiquity*, especially 4–7. The second pandemic was the early modern cycle (1347–1720) initiated by the Black Death. See Carmichael, "Bubonic Plague," 628–31. The third pandemic, in which bubonic plague spread worldwide beginning in the 1870s, continues today. See Echenberg, *Plague Ports*.

5. Carmichael, "Contagion Theory and Contagion Practice"; Henderson, "The Black Death in Florence."

6. Hays, "Historians and Epidemics"; Theilmann and Cate, "A Plague of Plagues"; Cunningham, "Identifying Disease in the Past"; Arrizabalaga, "Problematizing Retrospective Diagnosis."

7. Mitchell, "Retrospective Diagnosis."

8. Twigg, *The Black Death*, argued for anthrax; Scott and Duncan, *The Return of the Black Death*, argued for a hemorrhagic fever; Cohn, *The Black Death Transformed*, argued for "any disease other than the rat-based bubonic plague" (1).

9. Recent genomic work has revealed the presence of *Y. pestis*, and this remains an area of frequent discoveries. Among those historians who have previously argued in favor of identifying the early modern plague with true bubonic plague are Benedictow, *The Black Death*; Gottfried, *The Black Death*; and Ziegler, *The Black Death*. Numerous microbiological studies from recent years are eloquently and coherently reviewed in Little, "Plague Historians in Lab Coats." Among the recent biological studies are Bos et al., "A Draft Genome of *Yersinia pestis*"; Schuenemann

et al., "Targeted Enrichment of Ancient Pathogens"; Haensch et al., "Distinct Clones of *Yerinia pestis* Caused the Black Death"; Drancourt et al., "*Yersinia pestis* Orientalis in Remains of Ancient Plague Patients; Drancourt et al., "Detection of 400-Year-Old *Yersinia pestis* DNA in Human Dental Pulp"; Raoult et al., "Molecular Identification by 'Suicide PCR.'" Historians who previously opposed the identification of bubonic plague, and who offered a variety of circumstantial evidence in its disproval, include Twigg, *The Black Death*; Scott and Duncan, *The Return of the Black Death*; Cohn, *The Black Death Transformed*; Herlihy, *The Black Death and the Transformation of the West*; Lerner, "Fleas."

10. Cunningham, "Transforming Plague," 209–11; Arrizabalaga, "Problematizing Retrospective Diagnosis."

11. See Horrox, *The Black Death*; Byrne, *The Black Death*; Kelly, *The Great Mortality*; Cantor, *In the Wake of the Plague*. See also the discussion in Getz, "Black Death and the Silver Lining."

12. De' Mussis, *Historia de morbo*, in Horrox, *The Black Death*, 20.

13. Ziegler, *The Black Death*, 17.

14. Byrne, *Daily Life during the Black Death*, 3.

15. Rosen, *A History of Public Health*, 44–45.

16. See, for example, Cipolla's many works, including *Faith, Reason, and the Plague*; *Fighting the Plague in Seventeenth-Century Italy*; *Public Health and the Medical Profession in the Renaissance*; as well as Carmichael, *Plague and the Poor*; "Plague Legislation"; "Contagion Theory and Contagion Practice"; and Slack, *Impact of Plague* and "Responses to Plague."

17. Slack, *Impact of Plague*, 227–54.

18. Naphy, *Plagues, Poisons, and Potions*, 19.

19. Slack, *Impact of Plague*, 295–310.

20. See Baldwin, *Contagion and the State*; Slack, "Responses to Plague," 111–12.

21. See note 16 above.

22. Naphy, *Plagues, Poisons, and Potions*, 20.

23. The records from 1582 include a petition from a resident of Granada, who appealed his detainment by Seville's gate guards. Health commissioners not only were willing to hear his petition, but also subsequently sent a member to investigate health in that city. The petition to remove Granada from the list of infected towns was subsequently granted. See chap. 4.

24. Cipolla, *Public Health*, 12–16.

25. Carmichael, *Plague and the Poor*; Pullan, *Rich and Poor in Renaissance Venice*.

26. Cipolla, *Public Health*, 35.

27. Archivo Municipal de Sevilla (hereafter AMS), sección 13, siglo XVI, tomo 5, f. 3v.

28. AMS, sección 13, siglo XVI, tomo 5, f. 3v.

29. AMS, sección 13, siglo XVI, tomo 5, f. 27, "en esta dia murio un muy buen enfermero que no e sentido poco su falta por ser muy grande para los enfermos."

30. The 1582 records are in AMS, "Papeles Importantes" for the sixteenth century (section 13), in two bound volumes (vols. 5 and 6). The 1600 epidemic records are in "Escribanías del Cabildo" for the sixteenth century (section 3), vol. 7.

31. Ortíz de Zúñiga, *Anales eclesiásticos*, 4:113; Villalba, *Epidemiologia Española*, 1:117–20.

32. Vincent, "La peste Atlantica de 1596–1602"; Clark, *The European Crisis of the 1590s*; Biraben, *Les hommes et la peste*, appendix 3; Martin, *Plague?*

33. The events of the epidemic of 1581–82 in Seville have recently been highlighted by Cook and Cook in *The Plague Files*. An excellent recounting of the multiple crises (famine, plague, locust infestation, the royal billeting of foreign troops, explosion at a gunpowder factory) faced by the *Asistente* Don Fernando de Torres y Portugal, the Conde de Villar, it narrates the events of 1582 and offers firsthand voices in accounts taken directly from the city council records.

34. Calvi, *Histories of a Plague Year*, 22–27.

35. Archivo General de Simancas (hereafter AGS), Guerra Antigua (hereafter GA), tomo 12, fol. 66.

36. Barrera-Osorio, *Experiencing Nature*, 29–55.

37. López Pérez and Rey Bueno, "Simón de Tovar"; Gil, *Arias Montano*, 141–56; López Piñero et al., *Diccionario histórico*, vol. 2:69–72, 371–72; Guerra, *Nicolás Bautista Monardes*; Boxer, *Two Pioneers of Tropical Medicine*; López Piñero, *Ciencia y técnica*, 144; Goodman, *Power and Penury*, 238.

38. Calvi, *Histories of a Plague Year*, 1–12; Cipolla, *Public Health*, 39–42; Ballesteros Rodriguez, *La peste en Córdoba*, 88–98.

Chapter One

1. There are several good descriptions of the city in its greatest century, which may be consulted for further information. Morgado, *Historia de Sevilla* (1589), is a laudatory volume written by a parish priest who relocated to the "very famous city of Seville" (*muy famosa ciudad de Sevilla*) from the town of Alcántara. See also Montoto de Sedas, *Sevilla en el Imperio*, much of which is summarized in English in Pike, *Enterprise and Adventure*. A more recently written synthesis is available in Morales Padrón, *Historia de Sevilla*.

2. Edwards, *The Spain of the Catholic Monarchs*, 38–67; Kamen, *Philip of Spain*, 90–91.

3. Carande, *Carlos V y sus banqueros*, comes in with a low estimate of population, while Domínguez Ortiz, *The Golden Age of Spain*, gives the higher estimate. See also Perry, *Crime and Society*, 23; Sentaurens, "Seville dans la seconde moitie du XVIe siecle"; Collantes de Terán, *Sevilla en la baja edad media*, 135–87.

4. Pérez Moreda, *La crisis de mortalidad*.

5. Cook and Cook, *Plague Files*, examines how one sixteenth-century governor of the city, Don Fernando de Torres y Portugal, the Conde de Villar, managed in the face of repeated crises.

6. Mena, *Tradiciones y leyendas Sevillanas*, 9–12.

7. Fletcher, *Moorish Spain*, 86.

8. Montoto de Sedas, *Sevilla en el Imperio*, 13.

9. Morales Padrón, *Historia de Sevilla*, 169.

10. Montoto de Sedas, *Sevilla en el Imperio*, 14–17.

11. Lunenfeld, *Keepers of the City*, 14–23; Edwards, *The Spain of the Catholic Monarchs*, 54–59.

12. Edwards, *Christian Córdoba*, 27–28; Morales Padrón, *Historia de Sevilla*, 321–33; Domínguez Ortíz, *Historia de Sevilla*, 311–17.

13. Morales Padrón, *Historia de Sevilla*, 215.

14. Ladero Quesada, *Historia de Sevilla*, 165–78.

15. Morales Padrón, *Historia de Sevilla*, 217.

16. *Ordenanças de Sevilla*, f. 2v.

17. Peraza, *Justicia de Sevilla*, cited in Perry, *Crime and Society*, 13.

18. Morales Padrón, *Historia de Sevilla*, 218.

19. Ladero Quesada, *Historia de Sevilla*, 170–71.

20. Ibid., 172.

21. AMS, sección 3, tomo 7, no. 10.

22. AMS, sección 3, tomo 7, no. 9.

23. AMS, sección 3, tomo 7, nos. 11–12.

24. *Ordenanças*, f. 1–1v.

25. Morales Padrón, *Historia de Sevilla*, 211.

26. *Ordenanças*, f. 2v.

27. Ladero Quesada, *Historia de Sevilla*, 185.

28. See Villalba, *Epidemiologia Española*; Velázquez y Sánchez, *Anales epidemicos*; Morales Padrón, 321–33.

29. Ladero Quesada, *Historia de Sevilla*, 64.

30. Pike, *Aristocrats and Traders*, 9.

31. Morales Padrón, *Historia de Sevilla*, 31.

32. "Relación del contagio que padeció esta ciudad de Sevilla el año de 1649," in "Memorias de diferentes cosas sucedidas en esta Muy Noble y Muy Leal Ciudad de Sevilla," manuscript 84-7-21, Biblioteca Colombina, ff. 55–56.

33. Ladero Quesada, *Historia de Sevilla*, 52.

34. Borja Palomo, *Memoria histórico crítica*, lists 1590, 1592, 1593, 1595, 1596, 1603, 1608, 1618, 1626, 1633, 1642, and 1649 as years of significant flooding. Carmona García, *El sistema de la hospitalidad pública*, 110, lists 1507, 1510, 1523, 1543–45, 1554, 1562, 1583, 1586, 1590–96.

35. Lindemann, *Medicine and Society*, 10.

36. AMS, sección 13, siglo XVI, tomo 3, f. 26. See also the discussion in Carmona, *Crónica urbana del malvivir*, 124–29.

37. Cook and Cook, *Plague Files*, 52–55.

38. Montoto de Sedas, *Sevilla en el Imperio*, 18.

39. Carmona, *Crónica urbana del malvivir*.

40. Montoto de Sedas, *Sevilla en el Imperio*, 19–20.

41. AMS, sección 13, siglo XVII, tomo 4, nos. 57, 58.

42. Albardonedo Freire, "Las trazas y construcción"; Wunder, "Classical, Christian, and Muslim Remains."

43. Collantes de Terán, *Sevilla in la baja edad media*, 81.

44. Ibid., 81–82.

45. Montoto de Sedas, *Sevilla en el Imperio*, 16.

46. AMS, sección 10, 1624 (primera escribanía).

47. Losana Méndez, *La sanidad*, 19.

48. See Collantes de Terán, *Sevilla en la baja edad media*, 84. Payments to these city workers appear frequently in the city's financial records: AMS, sección 10.

49. AMS, sección 3, tomo 17, no. 1.

50. AMS, sección 4, tomo 11, no. 8, f. 18–18v.

51. AMS, sección 1, cpta. 8, no. 133.

52. AMS, sección 13, siglo XVI, tomo 3, no. 27.

53. AMS, sección 10, cpta. 8, no. 37; cpta. 20, no. 1; cpta. 20, no. 16; cpta. 23, nos. 59, 98.

54. AMS, sección 10, cpta. 12, no. 35.

55. AMS, sección 10, cpta. 22, no. 81.

56. AMS, sección 3, tomo 11, no. 73.

57. AMS, sección 3, tomo 7, no. 8.

Chapter Two

1. Boccaccio, *Decameron*, 50.

2. "Bubones, landres, carbunclos simples, y complicados, y unos tabardillos tan arrebatados, y violentos, que en dos dias, uno y medio, quarto de dia, e instantaneamente, se caian los hombres muertos." Francisco de Ruesta, "Memorias eclesiasticas y seculares de la Muy Noble y Muy Leal Ciudad de Sevilla copiadas en Sevilla año de 1698," manuscript 59-1-3, Biblioteca Colombina, f. 97.

3. Stearns, *Infectious Ideas*, 39.

4. Conrad, *Western Medical Tradition*, 192–93; Kinzelbach, "Infection, Contagion, and Public Health"; Carlin, *Imagining Contagion in Early Modern Europe*.

5. Although Juan de Aviñón wrote his treatise in 1419, it was later published by Nicolas Monardes in 1545, an indication of the longevity of its concepts. Chinchilla, *Anales históricos* 1:347–55; Hernández Morejon, *Historia bibliográphica*, 5:72–73.

6. AMS, sección 13, siglo XVI, tomo 5, f. 27.

7. AMS, sección 13, siglo XVI, tomo 5, f. 29.

8. Freilas, *Preservacion de peste*, 5.

9. See Horrox, *The Black Death*, 100–101, 158–206.

10. Sharpe, "Isidore of Seville," 57.

11. Nutton, "The Seeds of Contagion"; Conrad, *Western Medical Tradition*, 193.

12. Sharpe, 57.

13. Horrox, *The Black Death*, 184.

14. Conrad, *Western Medical Tradition*, 263; French, *Medicine before Science*, 158–66; Arrizabalaga, Henderson, and French, *The Great Pox*, 234–51; Stearns, *Infectious Ideas*.

15. Carmichael, "Contagion Theory and Contagion Practice."

16. Carmichael, *Plague and the Poor*, 90.

17. Pullen, "Plague and Perceptions of the Poor," 106–7.

18. Slack, *Impact of Plague*, 195.

19. AMS, sección 13, siglo XVI, tomo 5, f. 3.

20. "Relación del contagio," ff. 52–107. Additional manuscripts held in the Biblioteca Colombina contain the same or related accounts. See Morales Padrón, *Memorias de Sevilla*, 12–20.

21. "Relación del contagio," f. 54–54v.

22. On medieval efforts at categorization, see Brodman, *Charity and Welfare*, 4–7.

23. Cavallo, *Charity and Power in Early Modern Italy*, 14–15; Flynn, *Sacred Charity*, 83–84; Martz, *Poverty and Welfare in Habsburg Spain*, 7–13.

24. Arrizabalaga, "Poor Relief in Counter-Reformation Castile."

25. Perry, *Gender and Disorder*, 159–60.

26. AMS, sección 13, siglo XVI, tomo 5, f. 71.

27. AMS, sección 13, siglo XVI, tomo 5, ff. 69v–70.

28. AMS, sección 13, siglo XVI, tomo 5, f. 107.

29. AMS, sección 13, siglo XVI, tomo 6, ff. 83–93.

30. AMS, sección 13, siglo XVI, tomo 6, f. 85.

31. In testimonies from doctors the next month (May 1582), the doctors refer to themselves as having been ordered by the commission to carry out these duties, but it is not clear from these records whether they were paid to do so or simply ordered to. AMS, sección 13, siglo XVI, tomo 6, ff. 272–76.

32. Carmona lists years of famine in *Crónica urbana de malvivir*, 185. For a discussion of locusts in Seville 1579–80, see Cook and Cook, *The Plague Files*, 19–21.

33. For example AMS, sección 3, tomo 17; sección 13, tomo 4, no. 23; sección 10, 10 Marzo 1626.

34. Monteano, *Los navarros ante el hambre*, 161–64. For an overview of the wider Mediterranean trade in grain, see Braudel, *The Mediterranean and the Mediterranean World*, 1:570–606.

35. AMS, sección 3, tomo 17.

36. AMS, sección 3, tomo 4, no. 23.

37. Nieto de Piña, *Discurso Fisico Economico de la Harina de Trigo*.

38. Matossian, *Poisons of the Past*, 47–58.

39. AMS, sección 13, siglo XVI, tomo 5, f. 69.

40. Granjel, *La medicina española renacentista*, 41.

41. Clouse, *Medicine, Government, and Public Health*, 46.

42. There are numerous studies of plague treatises, see especially Sudhoff, "Pestschriften"; Singer, "Some Plague Tractates"; Jones, "Plague and Its Metaphors"; Keiser, "Two Medieval Plague Treatises."

43. See Ollero Pina, *La universidad de Sevilla*, 369; López Piñero, *Ciencia y técnica*, 59–62, 112–13; Griffin, *The Crombergers of Seville*.

44. See López Piñero, *Ciencia y técnica*, 138–40; Wilson Bowers, "Tradition and Innovation," 34–36.

45. Mercado first published the Latin treatise, *De natura et conditionibus, praeservatione, et curatione pestis* in Madrid in 1598. The following year he published *Libro en que se trata con claridad la naturaleza, causas, providencia, y verdaderan orden y modo de curar la enfermedad vulgar, y peste que estos años se ha divulgado por toda España*. Carreras Panchón, *La peste y los medicos*, 47.

46. Carreras Panchón, *La peste y los medicos*, 45–50. Hernández Morejón, *Historia bibliográphica*, 4:193–95. Zamudio de Alfaro, *Orden para la cura y preservacion de las secas y carbuncos*. Valdivia, *Tractado en el qual se explica la essencia y naturaleza de la enfermedad (que llaman landres) que a andado en Sevilla el año de 99 y 600.601*. Pérez de Herrera, *Dubitationes ad maligni, popularisque morbi*.

47. Carreras Panchón, *La peste y los medicos*, 49.

48. Saavedra, *Parecer . . . en que dice que el estado de la salud de Sevilla no es la peste*. See Hernandez Morejon, *Historia bibliográphica*, 4:165–66.

49. Monardes, *Primera y segunda y tercera partes de la historia medicinal de las cosas que se traen de nuestras Indias Occidentales que sirven en medicina*; Valdés, *De la utilidad de la sangria en las viruelas y otras enfermedades de los muchachos*, and *Disputa y averiguaciones de la enfermedad pestilente*, Hidalgo de Agüero, *Tesoro de la verdadera cirugia y via particular contra la comun.*

50. AMS, sección 13, siglo XVI, tomo 6, f. 84.

51. AMS, sección 13, siglo XVI, tomo 6, f. 85.

52. Wilson Bowers, "Tradition and Innovation"; Castaño Almendral, *La obra quirurgica de Bartolomé Hidalgo de Agüero.*

53. AMS, sección 13, siglo XVI, tomo 6, f. 86. Of the three, *modorra* is the term most difficult to identify, though it was a common diagnosis in the sixteenth century for illnesses associated often with fever and lethargy. See Cook, *Born to Die*, 55–56. *Tabardete* is accepted as referring to typhus, and *tercianas* as referring to tercian fever, or a form of malaria.

54. AMS, sección 13, siglo XVI, tomo 6, ff. 272–77.

55. AMS, sección 13, siglo XVI, tomo 6, f. 273.

56. AMS, sección 13, siglo XVI, tomo 6, f. 274 (*"en esta cibdad no ay enfermedad de peste aunque ay algunas enfermedades pestilenciales"*).

57. AMS, sección 13, siglo XVI, tomo 5, ff. 278–79. This is one of the few documents that refers directly to a notebook or file of records from the epidemic: "*el senor conde asistente mando se ponga en el cuaderno con los demas autos de peste.*"

58. AMS, sección 13, siglo XVI, tomo 5, f. 34.

59. AMS, sección 13, siglo XVI, tomo 5, f. 35.

60. AMS, sección 13, siglo XVI, tomo 5, f. 108.

61. See Morales Padrón, 322–33; Velázquez y Sánchez, *Anales Epidemicos*, 61–115; Villalba, *Epidemiologia Española*, 1:77–139.

62. Slack, *Impact of Plague*, 200.

63. Cipolla, *Public Health*, 47–51.

64. This argument was first and most strongly made by Cipolla, *Public Health*, 18–20, and *Fighting the Plague*, 3–6, but has carried through in nearly all works dealing with plague.

65. See Cipolla, *Public Health*, 11–66; Carmichael, *Plague and the Poor*, 108–26; Porter, *Health, Civilization, and the State*, 37–42.

66. See, for example, Naphy, *Plagues, Poisons, and Potions*, 14, 20; Cipolla, *Fighting the Plague*, 5. On the establishment of permanent health boards, see Cipolla, *Public Health.*

67. AMS, sección 13, siglo XVI, tomo 6, f. 75.

68. AMS, sección 13, siglo XVI, tomo 5, ff. 38v–39.

69. A similar system is noted for Milan in Carmichael, "Contagion Theory and Contagion Practice," 216.

70. AMS, sección 13, siglo XVI, tomo 5, f. 12.

71. AMS, sección 13, siglo XVI, tomo 5, f. 2.

72. For example, AMS, sección 13, tomo 5, f. 61; sección 3, tomo 7, no. 17, fol. 34.

73. For example, AMS, sección 13, tomo 5, ff. 76, 77–79v, 81–82, 83, 93, 103; sección 3, tomo 7, no. 17, ff. 36, 38, 41.

74. For example, AMS, sección 13, tomo 5, f. 91, 113; sección 3, tomo 7, no. 17, ff. 33, 38.

75. AMS, sección 13, siglo XVI, tomo 6, f. 76.

76. Several forms of communal religious response, including vows and processions, are discussed in Christian, *Local Religion in Sixteenth-Century Spain.*

77. Ortíz de Zúñiga, *Anales eclesiásticos*, 4:115.

78. Detailed descriptions of religious processions during the epidemic of 1649 may be found in the "Relación del contagio," ff. 52–107. See also AMS, Aguila, tomo 20.

79. AMS, sección 13, siglo XVI, tomo 5, fol. 2; sección 3, tomo 7, no. 17, f. 69.

80. AMS, sección 13, siglo XVI, tomo 6, f. 76v.

81. AMS, sección 13, siglo XVI, tomo 6, f. 79v.

82. AMS, sección 10, carpeta 160, nos. 34, 35.

83. AMS, sección 13, siglo XVI, tomo 6, ff. 83–93.

84. See, for example, Ortiz de Zúñiga, *Anales eclesiásticos*, 4:34.

85. AMS, sección 10, carpeta 160. This file contains extensive financial records from epidemics between 1599 and 1682. The bulk of the file is from 1599–1601 and reflects payment records for salaries, medicines, and other costs of running these hospitals, but does not contain any kind of patient records.

86. AMS, sección 13, siglo XVI, tomo 5, f. 35.

87. Harden, "Typhus, Epidemic," 1081. Harden cites a mortality rate of 5 to 25 percent for untreated typhus. In contrast, Carmichael, "Bubonic Plague," 629, cites a mortality rate for untreated plague from 60 percent to nearly 100 percent. This contrast in mortality was also noted by medical men at the time; see, for example, Bartolomé Hidalgo de Agüero, "Tratado decimo tercerio de peste" and "Tratado decimo quarto de tavardillo" in *Tesoro de la Verdadera Cirugia* (1654).

88. Archivo de la Diputación Provincial de Sevilla, Cinco Llagas. Notations for 1599, for example, may be found in leg. 111, fol. 14.

89. See, for example, AMS, sección 13, siglo XVI, tomo 6, f. 154.

90. See Ballesteros Rodríguez, *La peste en Córdoba*, 157–67; Fernández Álvarez, *Peste y supervivencia en Oviedo*, 31–46; "Informe sobre el estado sanitario de Alcalá de Henares" in Simón Díaz, *Relaciones breves*, 43–45.

Chapter Three

1. AMS, sección 13, siglo XVI, tomo 5, f. 99.

2. According to Villalba, the epidemic was widespread throughout Spain, and Seville also suffered an outbreak of smallpox in 1580: Villalba, *Epidemiologia Española*, 1:117; Ortiz de Zúniga, *Anales eclesiásticos*, 4:113. Velázquez y Sánchez, *Anales epidémicos*, 74, directly disputes Ortiz de Zúniga's assertion that this earlier epidemic affected the subsequent outbreak of plague and typhus in 1582.

3. Vassburg, *Land and Society*, xv. Vassburg provides an equivalence for the *arroba* as 3.32 gallons of oil or 4.26 gallons of wine.

4. AMS, sección 13, siglo XVI, tomo 5, ff. 99–101v.

5. AMS, sección 13, siglo XVI, tomo 5, f. 169.

6. AMS, sección 13, siglo XVI, tomo 5, f. 169v.

7. Sufficiently detailed records to show this are only available for the sixteenth and seventeenth centuries. At what point such a system of flexibility developed is therefore unclear, but likely extends earlier in time.

8. Amelang, *A Journal of the Plague Year*, 35.

9. Brockliss and Jones, *The Medical World of Early Modern France*, 40–41.

10. Cavallo, *Charity and Power*, 44–57.

11. For another study similarly indebted to Cavallo's interpretive framework, see Horden, "Ritual and Public Health," 17–40.

12. AMS, sección 13, siglo XVI, tomo 5, ff. 36–38; 41; 187–97.

13. It should be noted that neither document set of plague records contains evidence of petitions that were denied, which raises several questions. Part of the answer may lie in the fact that the two document sets are not catalogued together, but are found in separate sections of the archive ("Papeles Importantes" and "Escribanías del Cabildo"), which points toward a lack of cohesion in preservation. Given that both are incomplete it seems possible that such documents were filed separately at some time and subsequently lost. Despite this lack, the existence of such large numbers of petitions granted remains important and reflects the city's public health strategy.

14. AMS, sección 13, siglo XVI, tomo 5, f. 68.

15. AMS, sección 13, siglo XVI, tomo 6, ff. 2, 3.

16. AMS, sección 13, siglo XVI, tomo 6, f. 280.

17. AMS, sección 13, siglo XVI, tomo 6, f. 158.

18. AMS, sección 13, siglo XVI, tomo 5, f. 187.

19. For example, AMS, sección 13, siglo XVI, tomo 5, ff. 55, 169, 198, 227; tomo 6, f. 178.

20. AMS, sección 13, siglo XVI, tomo 5, ff. 169, 198.

21. AMS, sección 13, siglo XVI, tomo 5, f. 55.

22. AMS, sección 13, siglo XVI, tomo 5, f. 62.

23. AMS, sección 13, siglo XVI, tomo 5, f. 198.

24. AMS, sección 13, siglo XVI, tomo 5, f. 179.

25. AMS, sección 13, siglo XVI, tomo 5, f. 198v.

26. AMS, sección 13, siglo XVI, tomo 5, ff. 227–28.

27. AMS, sección 13, siglo XVI, tomo 6, f. 128.

28. AMS, sección 13, siglo XVI, tomo 6, f. 126.

29. AMS, sección 13, siglo XVI, tomo 6, ff. 127, 129.

30. AMS, sección 3, tomo 7, no. 17, ff. 73, 116–17.

31. AMS, sección 3, tomo 7, no. 17, ff. 73v, 118.

32. AMS, sección 13, siglo XVI, tomo 5, f. 136. Their petition is granted in f. 134v.

33. AMS, sección 13, siglo XVI, tomo 6, f. 136.

34. AMS, sección 3, tomo 7, no. 17, fol. 371.

35. See Pike, *Enterprise and Adventure*; Helen Nader, "Desperate Men, Questionable Acts," 404–5.

36. AMS, sección 13, siglo XVI, tomo 6, ff. 33–34v.

37. AGS, GA, leg. 126, no. 63.

38. AMS, seccíon 13, siglo XVI, tomo 6, ff. 265–69.

39. AMS, sección 13, siglo XVI, tomo 6, ff. 147, 155, 157, 159, 191, 194, 196, 198, 207, 265, 290, 306.

40. AMS, sección 3, tomo 7, no. 17, fol. 39.

41. AMS, sección 13, siglo XVI, tomo 5, f. 41; sección 3, tomo 7, f. 123.

42. AMS, sección 13, siglo XVI, tomo 5, f. 36; sección 3, tomo 7, no. 17, ff. 123, 182, 237, 268.

43. See for example, AMS, sección 13, siglo XVI, tomo 5, ff. 31, 76–77, 81, 83; sección 3, tomo 7, no. 17, ff. 35, 39, 115.

44. AMS, sección 13, siglo XVI, tomo 5, ff. 77, 81, 83, 91.

45. AMS, sección 13, siglo XVI, tomo 5, ff. 109, 160.

46. AMS, sección 3, tomo 7, no. 17, f. 115.

47. AMS, sección 13, siglo XVI, tomo 5, f. 266.

48. AMS, sección 13, siglo XVI, tomo 5, f. 199–99v.

49. AMS, sección 13, siglo XVI, tomo 5, ff. 188–91v, 197v.

50. AMS, sección 13, siglo XVI, tomo 5, ff. 192–94.

51. Toledo's interview of Tomás is contained in AMS, sección 13, siglo XVI, tomo 5, ff. 220–22; the letters carried by him are ff. 223–24.

52. AMS, sección 13, siglo XVI, tomo 5, ff. 217–22.

53. AMS, sección 13, siglo XVI, tomo 5, f. 204.

54. AMS, sección 13, siglo XVI, tomo 5, ff. 226, 234–35.

55. AMS, sección 13, siglo XVI, tomo 5, f. 52.

56. AMS, sección 13, siglo XVI, tomo 5, f. 52.

57. AMS, sección 13, siglo XVI, tomo 5, f. 53.

58. AMS, sección 13, siglo XVI, tomo 5, f. 54.

Chapter Four

1. Reher, *Town and Country in Pre-Industrial Spain*, 168.

2. Martz, *Poverty and Welfare*, 4.

3. AMS, sección 13, siglo XVI, tomo 5, f. 57.

4. For the distinction between cities, town, and villages, see Nader, *Liberty in Absolutism*, xv–xvi.

5. The story of Eyam and the epidemic of 1666 have been recounted often in poems and stories, and the town is now a popular tourist site. See the town website, www.eyamplaguevillage.co.uk. For a critical assessment of historical events versus myths of Eyam, see Wallis, "Dreadful Heritage."

6. AMS, sección 13, siglo XVI, tomo 5, f. 25.

7. AMS, sección 13, siglo XVI, tomo 5, ff. 6, 25.

8. AMS, sección 13, siglo XVI, tomo 5, f. 25–25v.

9. AMS, sección 13, siglo XVI, tomo 5, f. 26v.

10. AMS, sección 13, siglo XVI, tomo 5, ff. 6–7.

11. AMS, sección 13, siglo XVI, tomo 5, f. 69v.

12. See for example AMS, sección 13, siglo XVI, tomo 5, ff. 5–7, 134.

13. AMS, sección 13, siglo XVI, tomo 5, ff. 137, 256.

14. AMS, sección 13, siglo XVI, tomo 5, f. 3v.

15. AMS, sección 13, siglo XVI, tomo 5, f. 27.

16. AMS, sección 13, siglo XVI, tomo 5, f. 3v.

17. AMS, sección 13, siglo XVI, tomo 5, f. 4v.

18. AMS, sección 3, tomo 7, no. 17, f. 515.

19. AMS, sección 3, tomo 7, no. 17, ff. 36–38.
20. AMS, sección 13, siglo XVI, tomo 5, f. 256.
21. Morgado, *Historia de Sevilla*, 41.
22. AMS, sección 13, siglo XVI, tomo 5, f. 27.
23. AMS, sección 13, siglo XVI, tomo 5, f. 109.
24. Morgado, *Historia de Sevilla*, 41.
25. AMS, sección 13, siglo XVI, tomo 5, f. 62.
26. AMS, sección 13, siglo XVI, tomo 5, ff. 69–73v.
27. AMS, sección 13, siglo XVI, tomo 5, ff. 104, 171.
28. AMS, sección 13, siglo XVI, tomo 5, ff. 172–78.
29. AGS, Estado, leg. 184, no. 77.
30. AMS, sección 13, siglo XVI, tomo 5, f. 173.
31. AMS, sección 13, siglo XVI, tomo 5, f. 171, 179.
32. AMS, sección 13, siglo XVI, tomo 5, f. 179.
33. AMS, sección 13, siglo XVI, tomo 5, f. 238–38v.
34. AMS, sección 13, siglo, XVI, tomo 5, ff. 238–54.
35. AMS, sección 13, siglo XVI, tomo 5, f. 239.
36. AMS, sección 13, siglo XVI, tomo 5, f. 261.
37. AMS, sección 13, siglo XVI, tomo 5, f. 237.
38. AMS, sección 13, siglo XVI, tomo 6, f. 123–23v.
39. AMS, sección 13, siglo XVI, tomo 6, ff. 126–28v.
40. AMS, sección 13, siglo XVI, tomo 6, f. 127.
41. AMS, sección 13, siglo XVI, tomo 6, ff. 243–60.
42. AMS, sección 13, siglo XVI, tomo 6, ff. 248, 252.
43. See Clark, *The European Crisis of the 1590s*; Biraben, *Les hommes et la peste*, appendix 3; Martin, *Plague*.
44. AMS, sección 3, tomo 7, no. 17, ff. 69–71.
45. AMS, sección 3, tomo 7, no. 17, f. 74.
46. AMS, sección 3, tomo 7, no. 17, f. 75.
47. AMS, sección 3, tomo 7, no. 17, f. 85.
48. AMS, sección 3, tomo 7, no. 17, ff. 127–45, 148.
49. AMS, sección 3, tomo 7, no. 17, f. 148.
50. AMS, sección 3, tomo 7, no. 17, ff. 149, 161–64v.
51. AMS, sección 3, tomo 7, no. 17, f. 162v.
52. AMS, sección 3, tomo 7, no. 17, ff. 152–60v.
53. AMS, sección 3, tomo 7, no. 17, ff. 150v, 171.
54. AMS, sección 3, tomo 7, no. 17, f. 228.
55. AMS, sección 3, tomo 7, no. 17, ff. 176–79, 240–45.
56. AMS, sección 3, tomo 7, no. 17, ff. 180–81.
57. AMS, sección 3, tomo 7, no. 17, f. 201v.
58. AMS, sección 3, tomo 7, no. 17, f. 127.

Chapter Five

1. Villalba, *Epidemiologia Española*, 1:117–19; Velázquez y Sánchez, *Anales epidémicos*, 74.

2. AMS, sección 3, tomo 7, no. 10.

3. For example, see the extensive records in AGS, Estado, legs. 183, 184; and in AGS, Camara de Castilla.

4. AMS, sección 3, tomo 7, no. 9.

5. AMS, sección 3, tomo 7, nos. 11–12.

6. García-Ballester, McVaugh, and Rubio-Vela, *Medical Licensing and Learning in Fourteenth-Century Valencia.*

7. Feros, *Kingship and Favoritism*; Elliott, *The Count-Duke of Olivares.*

8. Brockliss and Jones, *Medical World of Early Modern France,* 350–52.

9. Muñoz Garrido and Muñiz Fernández, *Fuentes legales de la medicina española,* 17; Granjel, *La medicina española antigua y medieval,* 124.

10. Iborra, *Historia del protomedicato,* 9; Campos Díez, *El real tribunal del protomedicato castellano,* 19–25.

11. Iborra, *Historia del protomedicato,* 26.

12. López Piñero, "The Medical Profession in Sixteenth-Century Spain," 85–90.

13. Goodman, *Power and Penury,* 222–23.

14. Iborra, *Historia del protomedicato,* 28–29.

15. Goodman, *Power and Penury,* 223–29; Gentilcore, "'All That Pertains to Medicine,'" 121–42.

16. See Clouse, *Medicine, Government, and Public Health.*

17. Clouse, "Administering and Administrating Medicine,"188–90; Goodman, *Power and Penury,* 217–19; Barrera-Osorio, "Local Herbs, Global Medicines," 163–81.

18. Clouse, "Administering and Administrating Medicine," 26.

19. AMS, sección 1, cpta. 174, no. 20; sección 3, tomo 11, no. 79; sección 4, tomo 22, f. 219.

20. Wilson Bowers, "Tradition and Innovation."

21. Betrán, *La peste en la Barcelona,* 320–23.

22. For such correspondence under Philip II, see AGS, GA, legs. 67, 100, 101, 109, 110, 112, 196.

23. Goodman, *Power and Penury,* 230–31.

24. AGS, GA, leg. 140, no. 46; Betrán, *La peste en la Barcelona,* 320.

25. Vincent, "La peste Atlantica de 1596–1602," 5–25.

26. Fernández Álvarez, *Peste y supervivencia en Oviedo*; Viñes Ibarrola, *Una epidemica de peste bubónica en el siglo XVI*; Monteano, *La ira de Dios*; Ballesteros Rodríguez, *La peste en Córdoba.*

27. For northern Spain, see Bennassar, *Recherches.* See also Fernández Álvarez, *Peste y supervivencia en Oviedo.* In Seville's municipal archive, the financial records alone from this epidemic run over eight hundred pages. AMS, sección 2, carpeta 160.

28. Bennassar, *Recherches,* 105–88.

29. Bennassar relies on this correspondence and reprints many of these documents. The bulk of this correspondence may be found in AGS, Estado, legs. 183, 184.

30. Carreras Panchón, *La peste y los medicos,* 45–48; Hernández Morejón, *Historia bibliográphica,* 3:83–86, 229; Chinchilla, *Anales históricos de la medicina,* 2:132–33, 139–46.

31. Zamudio de Alfaro, *Orden para la cura y preservacion de las secas y carbuncos* . . . , 2v.

32. Carreras Panchón, *La peste y los medicos*, 48–51, 153–60.

33. Barrera-Osoria, *Experiencing Nature*, 36.

34. Such correspondence during the reign of Philip II may be found throughout AGS, GA, including throughout leg. 109, 112, 113, 114, 126, 127.

35. AGS, GA, tomo 112, f. 65.

36. Archivo General de Indias, Indiferente, 1956, leg. 3, ff. 129–30. Similar warnings were also issued in later epidemics, see Archivo General de Indias, Indiferente, 436, leg. 14, ff. 332v–34v [1649]; 437, leg. 15, ff. 8v–9 [1649]; 441, leg. 29, ff. 163, 155v [1678].

37. AGS, GA, tomo 12, f. 66.

38. Cook and Cook, *Plague Files*, 61.

39. Ibid., 87.

40. Ibid., 91.

41. Ibid., 116–19.

42. See for example Archivo de la Real Chancillería de Valladolid, Salas de lo Civil, Escribanía de Fernando Alonso, Fenecidos, caja 1450, 8; Escribanía de Pérez Alonso, Olvidados, caja 1285, 10.

43. AGS, GA, leg. 112, nos. 70–71.

44. Cook and Cook, *Plague Files*, 98.

45. Fernández Álvarez, *Peste y supervivencia en Oviedo*, 50–51.

46. AMS, sección 3, tomo 7, f. 201v.

47. AMC, sección 9.05.01, caja 0848.

48. Nirenberg, *Communities of Violence*, 233–37; Horrox, *The Black Death*, 207–19; Naphy, *Plagues, Poisons, and Potions*, 4–5.

49. Manzoni, *The Column of Infamy*.

50. Riera and Jiménez Muñoz, "Avisos en España de la peste de Milan," 165–68; Betrán, 323–24.

51. Archivo Municipal de Córdoba, sección 9.05.01, caja 0848; AMS, secc. 4, Tomo 13, no. 78.

52. AMS, sección 4, siglo XVII, tomo 13, no. 86, fol. 252.

53. Slack, *Impact of Plague*, 201.

54. Brockliss and Jones, *Medical World*, 69, 351–52.

55. Granjel, *La medicina española del siglo XVIII*, 117–19; Varela Peris, "El papel de la Junta Suprema," 315–40.

56. Henderson, *London and the National Government*, 33–45.

57. A good example is the file in Córdoba's municipal archive relating to this epidemic, which runs to nearly three hundred folios, predominately official correspondence from the Junta.

58. Bradley, *The Plague at Marseilles Consider'd*.

59. AMS, sección 13, siglo XVIII, tomo 6, ff. 1–18.

60. See Varela Peris, "El papel de la Junta Suprema"; Hermosilla Molina, *Epidemia de fiebre amarilla*; Iglesias Rodríguez, *La epidemia gaditana de fiebre amarilla*; Carrillos and Ballester, *Enfermedad y sociedad*; Nadal, *La población española*.

Conclusion

1. For example, Campbell, *Black Death and Men of Learning*; McNeill, *Plagues and Peoples*; Bowsky, *The Black Death*. In the same vein, works such as Huppert, *After the Black Death*, take the Black Death as a reference point of change.

2. For example, Huppert, *After the Black Death*; Herlihy, *The Black Death and the Transformation of the West*.

3. These stories are most evident in the works of Cipolla, Calvi, and DeFoe.

4. DeFoe, *A Journal of the Plague Year*; Moote and Moote, *The Great Plague*; Jones, "Plague and Its Metaphors"; Bertrand, *A Historical Relation of the Plague at Marseille*.

Bibliography

List of Archives

Archivo de la Diputación Provincial de Sevilla
    Hospitales y Centros Benéficos
Archivo General de Indias
    Indiferente
Archivo General de Simancas (AGS)
    Estado
    Guerra Antigua (GA)
    Camara de Castilla
Archivo General de Carmona
    Sección 4: Beneficencia y Sanidad
Archivo Municipal de Córdoba
    Sección 9: Beneficiencia, Sanidad y Asistencia Social
Archivo Municipal de Loja
Archivo Municipal de Sevilla (AMS)
    Sección 1: Archivo de Privilegios
    Sección 2: Archivo de Contaduría
    Sección 3: Escribanías del Cabildo, siglo XVI
    Sección 4: Escribanías del Cabildo, siglo XVII
    Sección 10: Actas Capitulares
    Sección 11: Papeles del Conde de Aguila
    Sección 13: Papeles Importantes, siglo XVI
Archivo de la Real Chancillería de Valladolid
    Salas de lo Civil
        Escribanía de Fernando Alonso
            Fenecidos
            Olvidados
        Escribanía de Pérez Alonso
            Fenecidos
            Olvidados
Biblioteca Colombina

Published Sources

Albardonedo Freire, Antonio José. "Las trazas y construcción de la Alameda de Hércules." *Laboratorio de Arte* 11 (1998): 135–66.

————. *El urbanismo de Sevilla durante el reinado de Felipe II.* Sevilla: Guadalquivir Ediciones, 2002.

Amelang, James S., ed. and trans. *A Journal of the Plague Year: The Diary of the Barcelona Tanner Miquel Parets, 1651.* New York: Oxford University Press, 1991.

Amundsen, Darrel W. "Medical Deontology and Pestilential Disease in the Late Middle Ages." *Journal of the History of Medicine and Allied Sciences* 32, no. 4 (1977): 403–21.

Arrizabalaga, Jon. "La enfermedad y la asistencia hospitalaria." In *Historia de la ciencia y de la técnica en la corona de Castilla,* edited by Luis García Ballester, 603–29. Vol. 1. Valladolid: Junta de Castilla y León, 2002.

————. "Facing the Black Death: Perceptions and Reactions of University Medical Practitioners." In *Practical Medicine from Salerno to the Black Death,* edited by L. García-Ballester, R. K. French, J. Arrizabalaga, and A. Cunningham, 237–88. New York: Cambridge University Press, 1994.

————. "Poor Relief in Counter-Reformation Castile: An Overview." In *Health Care and Poor Relief in Counter-Reformation Europe,* edited by Ole Peter Grell, Andrew Cunningham, and Jon Arrizabalaga, 151–76. New York: Routledge, 1999.

————. "Problematizing Retrospective Diagnosis in the History of Disease." *Asclepio* 54, no. 1 (2002): 51–70.

Arrizabalaga, Jon, John Henderson, and Roger French, *The Great Pox: The French Disease in Renaissance Europe.* New Haven: Yale University Press, 1997.

"Avian Flu Timeline." *CBC News,* May 12, 2008. http://www.cbc.ca/news/background/avianflu/timeline.html.

Aviñón, Juan de. *Sevillana medicina.* 1545. Reprint, Sevilla: Sociedad de Bibliófilas Andalúces, 1885.

Baldwin, Peter. *Contagion and the State in Nineteenth-Century Europe.* New York: Cambridge University Press, 1999.

Ballesteros Rodríguez, Juan. *La peste en Córdoba.* Córdoba: Publicaciones de la Excma. Diputación Provincial, 1982.

Barrera-Osorio, Antonio. *Experiencing Nature: The Spanish American Empire and the Early Scientific Revolution.* Austin: University of Texas Press, 2006.

————. "Local Herbs, Global Medicines: Commerce, Knowledge, and Commodities in Spanish America." In *Merchants and Marvels: Commerce, Science, and Art in Early Modern Europe,* edited by Pamela H. Smith and Paula Findlen, 163–81. New York: Routledge, 2002.

Benedictow, Ole. *The Black Death, 1346–1353: The Complete History.* Woodbridge, UK: Boydell Press, 2004.

Bennassar, Bartolomé. *Recherches sur les grandes epidémies dans le nord de l'Espagne á la fin du XVIᵉ siécle: Problémes de documentation et de méthode.* Paris: S.E.V.P.E.N., 1969.

Betrán, José Luis. *La peste en la Barcelona de los Austrias.* Lleida: Editorial Milenio, 1996.

Betrán Moya, José Luis. "La consolidación de la vuitena del morbo en la ciudad de Barcelona (1560–1600)." *Pedralbes* 13, no. 1 (1993): 631–42.

Bertrand, Jean-Baptiste. *A Historical Relation of the Plague at Marseille in the Year 1720.* Translated by Anne Plumptre. 1805. Reprint, London: Gregg International, 1973.

Biraben, Jean Noel. *Les hommes et la peste en France et dans les pays européens et mediterranéens.* 2 vols. Paris: Mouton, 1975–76.

Bluestein, Greg. "Man in 2007 TB Scare Sues CDC over Privacy." *Denver Post,* April 30, 2009. http://www.denverpost.com/search/ci_12258920.

Boccaccio, Giovanni. *The Decameron.* Translated by G. H. McWilliam. New York: Penguin Classics, 1972.

Borja Palomo, Don Francisco de. *Memoria histórico crítica sobre las riadas ó grandes avenidas del Guadalquivir en Sevilla, desde principios del sigo XV hasta nuestros días.* Sevilla, 1887.

Bos, Kirsten I., Verena J. Schuenemann, G. Brian Golding, Hernán A. Burbano, Nicholas Waglechner, Brian K. Coombes, Joseph B. McPhee, Sharon W. DeWitte, Matthias Meyer, Sarah Schmedes, James Wood, David J. D. Earn, D. Ann Herring, Peter Bauer, Hendrik N. Poinar, and Johannes Krause. "A Draft Genome of *Yersinia pestis* from Victims of the Black Death." *Nature* 478, no. 7370 (2011): 506–10. http://dx.doi.org/10.1038/nature10549.

Bowsky, William M., ed. *The Black Death: A Turning Point in History?* New York: Holt, Rinehart, and Winston, 1971.

Boxer, C. R. *Two Pioneers of Tropical Medicine: García D'Orta and Nicolás Monardes.* London: Hispanic and Luso-Brazilian Councils, 1963.

Bradley, Richard. *The Plague at Marseilles Consider'd.* London, 1721. http://www.gutenberg.org/files/31807/31807-h/31807-h.htm.

Braudel, Fernand. *The Mediterranean and the Mediterranean World in the Age of Philip II.* Translated by Siân Reynolds. Vol. 1. 1949. Reprint, New York: Harper and Row, 1972.

Brockliss, Laurence and Colin Jones. *The Medical World of Early Modern France.* New York: Clarendon Press, 1997.

Brodman, James William. *Charity and Welfare: Hospitals and the Poor in Medieval Catalonia.* Philadelphia: University of Pennsylvania Press, 1998.

Byrne, Joseph P. *The Black Death.* Westport, CT: Greenwood Press, 2004.

———. *Daily Life during the Black Death.* Westport, CT: Greenwood Press, 2006.

Calvi, Giulia. *Histories of a Plague Year: The Social and the Imaginary in Baroque Florence.* Translated by Dario Biocca and Bryant T. Ragan, Jr. Berkeley and Los Angeles: University of California Press, 1989.

Campbell, Anna Montgomery. *The Black Death and Men of Learning.* New York: Columbia University Press, 1931.

Campos Díez, María Soledad. *El real tribunal del protomedicato castellano.* Cuenca: Universidad de Castilla-La Mancha, 1999.

Cantor, Norman. *In the Wake of the Plague: The Black Death and the World It Made.* New York: Harper Perenial, 2002.

Carande, Ramon. *Carlos V y sus banqueros: La vida económica en Castilla, 1516–1556.* Madrid: Revista de Occidente, 1943.

Carlin, Claire L., ed. *Imagining Contagion in Early Modern Europe.* New York: Palgrave, 2005.

Carmichael, Ann. "Bubonic Plague." In Kipple, *The Cambridge World History of Human Disease,* 628–31.

———. "Contagion Theory and Contagion Practice in Fifteenth-Century Milan." *Renaissance Quarterly* 44, no. 2 (1991): 213–56.

———. "Plague Legislation in the Italian Renaissance." *Bulletin of the History of Medicine* 57, no. 4 (1983): 508–25.

———. *Plague and the Poor in Renaissance Florence.* Cambridge: Cambridge University Press, 1986.

Carmona, Juan. *Tractatus de peste et febre cum punticulis.* Sevilla, 1588.

Carmona, Juan Ignacio. *Crónica urbana del malvivir (s. XIV–XVII): Insalubridad, desamparo y hambre en Sevilla.* Sevilla: Universidad de Sevilla, 2000.

Carmona García, Juan I. *El extenso mundo de la pobreza: La otra cara de la Sevilla imperial.* Sevilla: Ayuntamiento de Sevilla, 1993.

———. *La peste en Sevilla.* Sevilla: Ayuntamiento de Sevilla, 2004.

———. *El sistema de la hospitalidad pública en la Sevilla del antiguo régimen.* Sevilla: Diputación Provincial de Sevilla, 1979.

Carreras Panchón, Antonio. "Dos testimonios sobre la epidemia de peste de 1599 en Valladolid." *Asclepio* 25 (1973): 351–57.

———. *La peste y los medicos en la España del renacimiento (1475–1610).* Salamanca: Universidad de Salamanca, 1976.

Carrillos, Juan L., and Luis Garcia Ballester. *Enfermedad y sociedad en la Málaga de los siglos xviii y xix: La fiebre amarilla (1741–1821).* Málaga: Universidad de Málaga, 1980.

Castaño Almendral, Alfonso A. *La obra quirurgica de Bartolomé Hidalgo de Agüero.* Salamanca: Universidad de Salamanca, 1959.

Cavallo, Sandra. *Charity and Power in Early Modern Italy: Benefactors and Their Motives in Turin, 1541–1789.* New York: Cambridge University Press, 1995.

Centers for Disease Control and Prevention. "Update: Severe Acute Respiratory Syndrome—Toronto, Canada, 2003." *Morbidity and Mortality Weekly Report* 52, no. 23 (2003): 547–50. http://www.cdc.gov/mmwr/preview/mmwrhtml/mm5223a4.htm.

Chinchilla, Don Anastasio. *Anales históricos de la medicina en general y biográfico-bibliográficos de la española en particular.* 4 vols. 1845–46. Reprint, New York: Johnson Reprint Corporation, 1967. http://hicido.uv.es/morejon_Chinchilla/index.html.

Christian, William. *Local Religion in Sixteenth-Century Spain.* Princeton: Princeton University Press, 1981.

Cipolla, Carlo M. *Cristofano and the Plague: A Study in the History of Public Health in the Age of Galileo.* New York: Harper Collins, 1973.

———. *Faith, Reason, and the Plague: A Tuscan Story of the Seventeenth Century.* Translated by Muriel Kittel. Ithaca: Cornell University Press, 1979.

———. *Fighting the Plague in Seventeenth-Century Italy.* Madison: University of Wisconsin Press, 1981.

———. *Public Health and the Medical Profession in the Renaissance.* New York: Cambridge University Press, 1976.

Clark, Peter, ed. *The European Crisis of the 1590s.* London: George Allen & Unwin, 1985.

Clouse, Michele. "Administering and Administrating Medicine: Regulation of the Medical Marketplace in Philip II's Spain." PhD diss., University of California, Davis, 2004.

————. *Medicine, Government, and Public Health in Philip II's Spain: Shared Interests, Competing Authorities.* Burlington, VT: Ashgate, 2011.

Cohn, Samuel K., Jr. *The Black Death Transformed: Disease and Culture in Early Renaissance Europe.* New York: Oxford University Press, 2002.

————. *Cultures of Plague: Medical Thought at the End of the Renaissance.* New York: Oxford University Press, 2010.

Collantes de Terán Sánchez, Antonio. *Sevilla in la baja edad media: La ciudad y sus hombres.* Sevilla: Publicaciones del Ayuntamiento, 1977.

Conrad, Lawrence I., Michael Neve, Vivian Nutton, Roy Porter, and Andrew Wear. *The Western Medical Tradition.* New York: Cambridge University Press, 1995.

Cook, Alexandra Parma, and Noble David Cook. *The Plague Files: Crisis Management in Sixteenth-Century Seville.* Baton Rouge: Louisiana State University Press, 2009.

Cook, Noble David. *Born to Die: Disease and New World Conquest, 1492–1650.* New York: Cambridge University Press, 1998.

Cunningham, Andrew. "Identifying Disease in the Past: Cutting the Gordian Knot." *Asclepio* 54, no. 1 (2002): 13–34.

————. "Transforming Plague: The Laboratory and the Identity of Infectious Disease." In *The Laboratory Revolution in Medicine,* edited by Andrew Cunningham and Perry Williams, 209–44. New York: Cambridge University Press, 1992.

Cunningham, Andrew, and Ole Peter Grell. *Four Horsemen of the Apocalypse: Religion, War, Famine, and Death in Reformation Europe.* Cambridge: Cambridge University Press, 2000.

Debus, Allen G. "Paracelsus and the Delayed Scientific Revolution in Spain." In *Reading the Book of Nature: The Other Side of the Scientific Revolution,* edited by Allen G. Debus and Michael T. Walton, 147–62. Kirksville, MO: Sixteenth Century Society Journal Publishers, 1998.

Defoe, Daniel. *A Journal of the Plague Year.* 1722. Edited by Paula R. Backscheider. New York: W. W. Norton and Company, 1992.

De Lollis, Barbara, and Michelle Kessler. "False Alarm: Fliers on Detained Flight Cleared." *USA Today,* April 2, 2003. http://www.usatoday.com/travel/news/2003/2003-04-01-sjc-sars.htm.

Dols, Michael W. *The Black Death in the Middle East.* Princeton: Princeton University Press, 1977.

————. "The Comparative Communal Responses to the Black Death in Muslim and Christian Societies." *Viator* 5 (1974): 269–87.

————. "The Second Plague Pandemic and Its Recurrences in the Middle East: 1347–1894." *Journal of the Economic and Social History of the Orient* 22, no. 2 (1979): 162–89.

Domínguez Ortiz, Antonio. *The Golden Age of Spain, 1516–1659.* Translated by James Casey. New York: Basic Books, 1971.

Drancourt, Michel, Gérard Aboudharam, Michel Signoli, Olivier Dutour, and Didier Raoult. "Detection of 400-Year-Old *Yersinia pestis* DNA in Human Dental Pulp: An Approach to the Diagnosis of Ancient Septicemia." *PNAS* 95, no. 21 (1998): 12637–40. http://dx.doi.org/10.1073/pnas.95.21.12637.

Drancourt, Michel, and Didier Raoult. "Molecular Detection of *Yersinia pestis* in Dental Pulp." *Microbiology* 150, no. 2 (2004): 263–64. http://dx.doi.org/10.1099/mic.0.26885-0.

Drancourt, Michel, Michel Signoli, La Vu Dang, Bruno Bizot, Véronique Roux, Stéfan Tzortzis, and Didier Raoult, "*Yersinia pestis* Orientalis in Remains of Ancient Plague Patients." *Emerging Infectious Diseases* 13, no. 2 (2007): 332–33.

Drexler, Madeline. *Emerging Epidemics: The Menace of New Infections.* New York: Penguin Books, 2009.

Edwards, John. *Christian Córdoba. The City and Its Region in the Late Middle Ages.* New York: Cambridge University Press, 1982.

———. *The Spain of the Catholic Monarchs, 1474–1520.* Malden, MA: Blackwell Publishing, 2000.

Elliott, J. H. *The Count-Duke of Olivares: The Statesman in an Age of Decline.* New Haven: Yale University Press, 1989.

Emery, Richard W. "The Black Death of 1348 in Perpignan." *Speculum* 42, no. 4 (1967): 611–23.

Fernández Álvarez, José Manuel. *Peste y supervivencia en Oviedo (1598–1599).* Oviedo: KRK Ediciones, 2003.

Fernández-Carrión, Mercedes, and José Luis Valverde. *Farmacia y sociedad en Sevilla en el siglo XVI.* Sevilla: Ayuntamiento de Sevilla, 1985.

Feros, Antonio. *Kingship and Favoritism in the Spain of Philip III, 1598–1621.* New York: Cambridge University Press, 2006.

Fletcher, Richard. *Moorish Spain.* Berkeley and Los Angeles: University of California Press, 1992.

Flynn, Maureen. *Sacred Charity: Confraternities and Social Welfare in Spain, 1400–1700.* Ithaca: Cornell University Press, 1989.

Fragoso, Juan. *Tratado de cirugia, sacado de la cirugia universal, que escrivió el Licenciado Juan Fragoso, conforme se practica en el Hospital General de Madrid.* Madrid, 1672.

Franco, Francisco. *Libro de las enfermedades contagiosas y de la preservacion dellas.* Sevilla, 1569.

Freilas (Freylas), Alonso de. *Preservacion de peste y curacion de ella.* Jaen, 1605.

French, Roger. *Medicine before Science.* New York: Cambridge University Press, 2003.

French, R., J. Arrizabalaga, A. Cunningham, and L. García-Ballester, eds., *Medicine from the Black Death to the French Disease.* Aldershot: Ashgate, 1998.

García-Ballester, Luis, ed. *Historia de la ciencia y de la técnica en la corona de Castilla.* 4 vols. Valladolid: Junta de Castilla y León, 2002.

———. "La producción y circulación de obras medicas." In *Historia de la ciencia y de la técnica en la corona de Castilla,* edited by Luís García Ballester, 709–88. Vol. 1. Valladolid: Junta de Castilla y León, 2002.

García-Ballester, Luis, Michael R. McVaugh, and Agustín Rubio-Vela. *Medical Licensing and Learning in Fourteenth-Century Valencia.* Philadelphia: The American Philosophical Society, 1989.

García-Ballester, Luis, Roger French, Jon Arrizabalaga, and Andrew Cunningham, eds. *Practical Medicine from Salerno to the Black Death.* New York: Cambridge University Press, 1994.

Garrett, Laurie. *The Coming Plague: Newly Emering Diseases in a World Out of Balance.* New York: Penguin Books, 1994.

Garza, Randall P. *Understanding Plague: The Medical and Imaginative Texts of Medieval Spain.* New York: Peter Lang, 2008.

Gentilcore, David. "'All That Pertains to Medicine': *Protomedici* and *Protomedicati* in Early Modern Italy" *Medical History* 38, no. 2 (1994): 121–42.

Gestoso y Pérez, José. *Curiosidades antiguas Sevillanas.* Sevilla, 1910.

Getz, Faye. "Black Death and the Silver Lining: Meaning, Continuity, and Revolutionary Change in Histories of Medieval Plague." *Journal of the History of Biology* 24, no. 2 (1991): 265–89.

Gil, Juan. *Arias Montano en su entorno: (Bienes y herederos).* Mérida: Editora Regional de Extremadura, 1998.

González Díaz, Antonio Manuel. *Poder urbano y asistencia social: El Hospital de San Hermenegildo de Sevilla (1453–1837).* Sevilla: Diputacion de Sevilla, 1997.

González Muñoz, María del Carmen. "Epidemias y enfermedades en Talavera de la Reina (ss. XVI y XVII)." *Hispania* 126 (1974): 149–68.

Goodman, David C. *Power and Penury: Government, Technology, and Science in Philip II's Spain.* New York: Cambridge University Press, 1988.

Gottfried, Robert. *The Black Death: Natural and Human Disaster in Medieval Europe.* New York: The Free Press, 1983.

Goubert, Jean-Pierre. "The Art of Healing: Learned Medicine and Popular Medicine in the France of 1790." Translated by Elborg Forster and Patricia M. Ranum. In *Medicine and Society in France: Selections from the Annales Economies, Sociétés, Civilisations,* edited by Robert Forster and Orest Ranum, 1–23. Vol. 6. Baltimore: Johns Hopkins University Press, 1980.

Granjel, Luis S. *La medicina española antigua y medieval.* Salamanca: Universidad de Salamanca, 1981.

———. *La medicina española renacentista.* Salamanca: Universidad de Salamanca, 1980.

Greenberg, Stephen. "Plague, the Printing Press, and Public Health in Seventeenth-Century London." *Huntington Library Quarterly* 67, no. 4 (2004): 509–27.

Grell, Ole Peter. "Conflicting Duties: Plague and the Obligations of Early Modern Physicians towards Patients and Commonwealth in England and the Netherlands." In *Doctors and Ethics: The Earlier Historical Setting of Professional Ethics,* edited by Andrew Wear, Johanna Geyer-Kordesch, and Roger French, 131–52. New York: Rodopoi, 1993.

Grell, Ole Peter, Andrew Cunningham, and Jon Arrizabalaga, eds. *Health Care and Poor Relief in Counter-Reformation Europe.* New York: Routledge, 1999.

Griffin, Clive. *The Crombergers of Seville: The History of a Printing and Merchant Dynasty.* Oxford: Clarendon Press, 1988.

Guerra, Francisco. *Nicolás Bautista Monardes: Su vida y su obra.* Mexico: D. F. Compañía fundidora de fierro y acero de Monterrey, 1961.

Guichot y Parody, D. Joaquin. *Historia del Excellentisimo Ayuntamiento de la Muy Noble, Muy Leal, Muy Heróica é Invicta Ciudad de Sevilla.* Sevilla: La Región, 1897.

Haensch, Stephanie, Raffaella Bianucci, Michel Signoli, Minoarisoa Rajerison, Michael Schultz, Sacha Kacki, Marco Vermunt, Darlene A. Weston, Derek Hurst, Mark Achtman, Elisabeth Carniel, Barbara Bramanti. "Distinct Clones of *Yersinia pestis* Caused the Black Death." *PloS Pathogens* 6 (October 2010). http://dx.doi.org/10.1371/journal.ppat.1001134.

Hammond, Mitchell Lewis. "Contagion, Honour, and Urban Life in Early Modern Germany." In Carlin, *Imagining Contagion in Early Modern Europe,* 94–106.

Hanska, Jussi. *Strategies of Sanity and Survival: Religious Responses to Natural Disasters in the Middle Ages.* Helsinki: Finnish Literature Society, 2002.

Harden, Victoria A. "Typhus, Epidemic." In Kiple, *The Cambridge World History of Human Disease,* 1080–84.

Hays, Jo N. "Historians and Epidemics: Simple Questions, Complex Answers." In Little, *Plague and the End of Antiquity,* 33–56.

Henderson, Alfred James. *London and the National Government, 1721–1742.* Durham: Duke University Press, 1945.

Henderson, John. "The Black Death in Florence: Medical and Communal Responses." In *Death and Towns: Urban Responses to the Dying and the Dead, 100–1600,* edited by Stephen Bassett, 136–47. Leicester: Leicester University Press, 1992.

———. "Epidemics in Renaissance Florence: Medical Theory and Government Response." In *Maladies et société (XII–XVIII siècles): Actes du colloque de Bielefeld, Novembre 1986,* edited by Neithard Bulst and Robert Delort, 165–84. Paris: Éditions du Centre National de la Recherche Scientifique, 1989.

Herlihy, David. *The Black Death and the Transformation of the West.* Edited by Samuel K. Cohn, Jr. Cambridge: Harvard University Press, 1997.

Hermosilla Molina, Antonio. *Epidemia de fiebre amarilla en Sevilla en el año 1800.* Sevilla: Talleres Gráficos, 1978.

Hernández Morejón, Don Antonio. *Historia bibliográphica de la medicina española.* 7 vols. 1842–52. Reprint, New York: Johnson Reprint Corporation, 1967. http://hicido.uv.es/morejón_Chinchilla/index.html.

Herrera, María Teresa, ed. *Diccionario español de textos medicos antiguos.* Vols. 1 and 2. Madrid: Arco/Libros, 1996.

Herrera Dávila, Joaquín. "Apología sevillana del aceite de Aparicio" *Archivo Hispalense* 91, nos. 276–78 (2008): 77–92.

———. *El Hospital del Cardenal de Sevilla y el Doctor Hidalgo de Agüero: Visión historicsanitaria del Hospital de San Hermenegildo (1455–1837).* Sevilla: Ediciones de la Fundación de Cultura Andaluza, 2010.

Herrera Dávila, Joaquín, and José Joaquín Jadraque Sánchez. "El *Tractatus de Curatione* (1606) de Juan de Sosa Sotomayor." *Archivo Hispalense* 91, nos. 276–78 (2008): 93–129.

Hidalgo de Agüero, Bartolomé. *Tesoro de la verdadera cirvgia y via particular contra la comun.* 1604. Reprint, Valencia, 1654.

Horden, Peregrine. "Ritual and Public Health in the Early Medieval City." In *Body and City: Histories of Urban Public Health,* edited by Sally Sheard and Helen Power, 17–40. Burlington, VT: Ashgate, 2000.

Horrox, Rosemary. *The Black Death.* Manchester: Manchester University Press, 1994.

Huppert, George. *After the Black Death: A Social History of Early Modern Europe.* Bloomington: Indiana University Press, 1998.

Iborra, D. Pasqual. "Memoria sobre la institucion del real proto-medicato." *Anales de la Real Academia de Medicina,* 1885–86. Reprinted as *Historia del protomedicato en España, 1477–1822.* Introduction and indexes by Juan Riera and Juan Granda-Juesas. Valladolid: Universidad de Valladolid, 1987.

Iglesias Rodríguez, Juan José. *La epidemia gaditana de fiebre amarilla de 1800.* Cádiz: Diputación de Cádiz, 1987.

Jones, Colin. "Plague and Its Metaphors in Early Modern France." *Representations*, no. 53 (Winter 1996): 97–127.

Jones, Kate E., Nikkita G. Patel, Marc A. Levy, Adam Storeygard, Deborah Balk, John L. Gittleman, and Peter Daszak. "Global Trends in Emerging Infectious Diseases." *Nature* 451, no. 7181 (2008): 990–94. http://dx.doi.org/10.1038/nature06536.

Keiser, George R. "Two Medieval Plague Treatises and Their Afterlife in Early Modern England." *Journal of the History of Medicine* 58, no. 3 (2003): 292–324.

Kelly, John. *The Great Mortality: An Intimate History of the Black Death, the Most Devastating Plague of All Time*. New York: HarperCollins, 2005.

Kilbourne Matossian, Mary. *Poisons of the Past: Molds, Epidemics, and History*. New Haven: Yale University Press, 1989.

Kinzelbach, Anne Marie. "Infection, Contagion, and Public Health in Late Medieval and Early Modern German Imperial Towns." *Journal of the History of Medicine and Allied Sciences* 61, no. 3 (2006): 369–89.

Kiple, Kenneth F., ed. *The Cambridge World History of Human Diseases*. Cambridge: Cambridge University Press, 1993.

Kottek, Samuel S., and Luis García-Ballester, eds. *Medicine and Medical Ethics in Medieval and Early Modern Spain: An Intercultural Approach*. Jerusalem: The Magnes Press, 1996.

Ladero Quesada, Miguel Angel. *Historia de Sevilla: La ciudad medieval (1248–1492)*. Sevilla: Universidad de Sevilla, 1989.

Lerner, Robert E. "Fleas: Some Scratchy Issues Concerning the Black Death." *Journal of The Historical Society* 8, no. 2 (2008): 205–28.

Lindemann, Mary. *Medicine and Society in Early Modern Europe*. New York: Cambridge University Press, 1999.

Little, Lester K., ed. *Plague and the End of Antiquity: The Pandemic of 541–750*. New York: Cambridge University Press, 2007.

———. "Plague Historians in Lab Coats." *Past and Present*, no. 213 (November 2011): 267–90.

López Pérez, Miguel and Mar Rey Bueno. "Simón de Tovar (1528–1596): redes familiars, naturaleza americana y comercio de maravillas en la Sevilla del XVI" *Dynamis* 26 (2006): 69–91.

López Piñero, José María. *Ciencia y técnica en la sociedad española de los siglos XVI y XVII*. Barcelona: Labor Universitaria, 1979.

———. "The Medical Profession in Sixteenth-Century Spain." In Russell, *The Town and State Physician in Europe*, 85–98.

———. "Paracelsus and His Work in Sixteenth- and Seventeenth-Century Spain." *Clio Medica* 8 (1973): 113–41.

López Piñero, José M., Thomas F. Glick, Víctor Navarro Brotóns, and Eugenio Portela Marco, eds. *Diccionario histórico de la ciencia moderna en España*. 2 vols. Madrid: Ediciones Península, 1983.

López Terrada, María Luz. "Los estudios historicomédicos sobre el Tribunal del protomedicato y las profesiones y ocupaciones sanitarias en la monarquía hispánica durante los siglos XVI al XVIII." *Dynamis* 16 (1996): 21–42.

López Terrada, María Luz, and Álvar Martínez Vidal. "El Tribunal del real protomedicato en la monarchía hispánica, 1593–1808." *Dynamis* 16 (1996): 17–20.

Losana Méndez, José. *La sanidad en la época del descubrimiento de América.* Madrid: Ediciones Cátedra, 1994.

Lunenfeld, Marvin. *Keepers of the City: The Corregidores of Isabella I of Castile (1474–1504).* New York: Cambridge University Press, 1987.

Martin, A. Lynn. *Plague?: Jesuit Accounts of Epidemic Disease in the Sixteenth Century.* Kirksville, MO: Sixteenth Century Journal Publishers, 1996.

Martínez Shaw, Carlos, ed. *Sevilla, siglo XVI: El corazón de las riquezas del mundo.* Madrid: Alianza Editorial, 1993.

Martz, Linda. *Poverty and Welfare in Habsburg Spain: The Example of Toledo.* Cambridge: Cambridge University Press, 1983.

McNeill, William H. *Plagues and Peoples.* New York: Doubleday, 1976.

Mena, José María de. *Tradiciones y leyendas Sevillanas.* Barcelona: Plaza y Janés Editores, 1994.

Mercado, Luis. *De natura et conditionibus, praeservatione, et curatione pestis.* Madrid, 1598.

———. *Libro en que se trata con claridad la naturaleza, causas, providencias, y verdaderan orden y modo de curar la enfermedad vulgar, y peste que en estos años se ha divulgado por toda España.* Madrid, 1599.

Mitchell, Piers D. "Retrospective Diagnosis and the Use of Historical Texts for Investigating Disease in the Past." *International Journal of Paleopathology* 1, no. 2 (2011): 81–88. http://dx.doi.org/10.1016/j.ijpp.2011.04.002.

Monardes, Nicolás. *Primera y segunda y tercera partes de la historia medicinal de las cosas que se traen de nuestras Indias Occidentales que sirven en medicina.* Sevilla, 1574.

Monteano, Peio J. *La ira de Dios: Los navarros en la era de la peste (1348–1723).* Pamplona: Pamiela, 2002.

———. *Los navarros ante el hambre, la peste, la guerra y la fiscalidad: Siglos XV y XVI.* Pamplona: Universidad Pública de Navarra, 1999.

Montoto de Sedas, Santiago. *Sevilla en el imperio (siglo XVI).* Sevilla: Nueva Librería, 1938.

Moote, A. Lloyd, and Dorothy C. Moote. *The Great Plague.* Baltimore: Johns Hopkins University Press, 2004.

Morales Padrón, Francisco. *Historia de Sevilla: La ciudad del quinientos.* Sevilla: Universidad de Sevilla, 1989.

———, ed. *Memorias de Sevilla (1600–1678).* Córdoba: Publicaciones del Monte de Piedad y Caja de Ahorros de Córdoba, 1981.

Moreno Toral, Esteban. *Estudio social y farmacoterapéutico de la lepra: El Hospital de San Lázaro de Sevilla (s. XIII–XIX).* Sevilla: Diputación de Sevilla, 1997.

Morgado, Alonso. *Historia de Sevilla en la qual se contienen sus antiguedades, grandezas, y cosas memorables en ella acontecidas, desde su fundacion hasta nuestros tiempos.* Sevilla, 1587.

Muñoz Garrido, Rafael, and Carmen Muñiz Fernández. *Fuentes legales de la medicina española (siglos XIII–XIX).* Salamanca: Universidad de Salamanca, 1969.

Nadal, Jordi. *Bautismos, desposorios y entierros: Estudios de historia demográfica.* Barcelona: Editorial Ariel, 1992.

———. *La población española, siglos XVI a XX.* Barcelona: Ariel, 1984.

Nader, Helen. "Desperate Men, Questionable Acts: The Moral Dilemma of Italian Merchants in the Spanish Slave Trade." *The Sixteenth Century Journal* 33, no. 2 (2002): 401–22.

———. *Liberty in Absolutist Spain: The Habsburg Sale of Towns, 1516–1700.* Baltimore: Johns Hopkins University Press, 1990.

Naphy, William G. *Plagues, Poisons, and Potions: Plague-Spreading Conspiracies in the Western Alps, c. 1530–1640.* Manchester: Manchester University Press, 2002.

Nieto de Piña, Don Christobal Jacinto. *Discurso Físico Economico de la Harina de Trigo, su conservacion y metodo para discernir la buena de la mala. Leida en la Real Sociedad de Medicina, y demas ciencias de Sevilla . . . 1781.* Sevilla: Real Sociedad de Medicina, 1784.

Nirenberg, David. *Communities of Violence: Persecution of Minorities in the Middle Ages* Princeton: Princeton University Press, 1996.

Nutton, Vivian. "Did the Greeks Have a Word for It?" In *Contagion: Perspectives from Pre-Modern Societies,* edited by Lawrence I. Conrad and D. Wujastyk, 137–62. Aldershot: Ashgate, 2000.

———, ed. *Pestilential Complexities: Understanding Medieval Plague.* London: The Wellcome Trust, 2008.

———. "The Seeds of Contagion: An Explanation of Contagion and Infection from the Greeks to the Renaissance." *Medical History* 27, no. 1 (1983): 1–34.

Ollero Pina, José Antonio. *La universidad de Sevilla en los siglos XVI y XVII.* Sevilla: Universidad de Sevilla, 1993.

Ordenanças de Sevilla: Recopilacion de las Ordenanças de la Muy Noble y Muy Leal Ciudad de Sevilla . . . Sevilla: Andres Grande, 1632.

Ortíz de Zúñiga, Diego. *Anales eclesiásticos y seculares de la Muy Noble y Muy Leal Ciudad de Sevilla.* 1677. Reprint, 5 vols., Madrid, 1796.

Peráza, Luis. *Justicia de Sevilla: Historia de esta ciudad.* Sevilla, n.d. (ca. 1650).

Pérez de Herrera, Cristóbal. *Discursos del Amparo de los legitimos pobres.* Madrid, 1598.

———. *Dubitationes ad maligni, popularisque morbi.* Madrid, 1599.

Pérez Moreda, Vicente. *Las crisis de mortalidad en al España interior (siglos XVI–XIX).* Madrid: Siglo Veintiuno de España Editors, 1980.

———. "The Plague in Castile at the End of the Sixteenth Century and Its Consequences." In *The Castilian Crisis of the Seventeenth Century,* edited by I. A. A. Thompson and Bartolomé Yun Casalilla, 32–59. Cambridge: Cambridge University Press, 1994.

Perry, Mary Elizabeth. *Crime and Society in Early Modern Seville.* Hanover: University Press of New England, 1980.

———. *Gender and Disorder in Early Modern Seville.* Princeton: Princeton University Press, 1990.

Phillips, William. "Peste Negra: The Fourteenth-Century Plague Epidemics in Iberia." In *On the Social Origins of Medieval Institutions: Essays in Honor of Joseph F. O'Callaghan,* edited by Donald J. Kagay and Theresa M. Vann, 47–62. Boston: Brill, 1998.

Pike, Ruth. *Aristocrats and Traders: Sevillian Society in the Sixteenth Century.* Ithaca: Cornell University Press, 1972.

———. *Enterprise and Adventure: The Genoese in Seville and the Opening of the New World.* Ithaca: Cornell University Press, 1966.

Platt, Colin. *King Death: The Black Death and Its Aftermath in Late Medieval England.* Toronto: University of Toronto Press, 1996.

Porter, Dorothy. *Health, Civilization, and the State: A History of Public Health from Ancient to Modern Times.* New York: Routledge, 1999.

Puerto, Javier. *La leyenda verde: Naturaleza, sanidad y ciencia en la corte de Felipe II (1527–1598).* Valladolid: Junta de Castilla y León, 2003.

Pullen, Brian. "Plague and Perceptions of the Poor in Early Modern Italy." In *Epidemics and Ideas*, edited by Terence Ranger and Paul Slack, 101–23. New York: Cambridge University Press, 1992.

———. *Rich and Poor and Renaissance Venice.* Cambridge: Harvard University Press, 1971.

Quammen, David. *Spillover.* New York: W. W. Norton and Company, 2012.

Raoult, Didier, Gérard Aboudharam, Eric Crubézy, Georges Larrouy, Bertrande Ludes, and Michel Drancourt. "Molecular Identification by 'Suicide PCR' of *Yersinia pestis* as the Agent of Medieval Black Death." *PNAS* 97, no. 23 (2000): 12800–803. http://dx.doi.org/10.1073/pnas.220225197.

Reher, David Sven. *Town and Country in Pre-Industrial Spain: Cuenca 1550–1870.* Cambridge: Cambridge University Press, 1990.

Riera, Juan, and J. M. Jiménez Muñoz. "Avisos en España de la peste de Milan." *Asclepio* 25 (1973): 165–68.

Rosen, George. *A History of Public Health.* 1958. Expanded ed. Baltimore: Johns Hopkins University Press, 1993.

Russell, Andrew W., ed. *The Town and State Physician in Europe from the Middle Ages to the Enlightenment.* Wolfenbüttel: Herzog August Bibliothek, 1981.

Saavedra, Juan de. *Parecer . . . en que dice que el estado de la salud de Sevilla no es la peste.* Sevilla, 1599.

Sánchez de Oropesa, Francisco. *Tratado de peste.* Sevilla, 1569.

———. *Tres proposiciones . . . a la ciudad de Sevilla, en que se ponen algunas advertencias para la preservación i cura del mal que anda en la ciudad.* Sevilla, 1599.

Schuenemann, Verena J., Kirsten Bos, Sharon DeWitte, Sarah Schmedes, Joslyn Jamieson, Alissa Mittnik, Stephen Forrest, Brian K. Coombes, James W. Wood, David J. D. Earn, William White, Johannes Krause, and Hendrik Poinar. "Targeted Enrichment of Ancient Pathogens yielding the pPCP1 Plasmid of *Yersinia pestis* from Victims of the Black Death." *PNAS* 108, no. 38 (2011): E746–52. http://dx.doi.org/10.1073/pnas.1105107108.

Scott, Susan, and Christopher Duncan. *Return of the Black Death.* John Wiley & Sons, 2004.

Sentaurens, Jean. "Seville dans la seconde moitie du XVIe siècle." *Bulletin Hispanique* 77, nos. 3–4 (1975): 321–90.

Sharpe, William D., ed. and trans. "Isidore of Seville: The Medical Writings." *Transactions of the American Philosophical Society.* Vol. 54, pt. 2. Philadelphia: The American Philosophical Society, 1964.

Simón Díaz, José, ed. *Relaciones breves de actos públicos celebrados en Madrid de 1541 a 1650.* Madrid: Instituto de Estudios Madrileños, 1982.

Singer, Dorothea Waley. "Some Plague Tractates (Fourteenth and Fifteenth Centuries)." *Proceedings of the Royal Society of Medicine* 9 (1916): 159–212.

ᴄlack, Paul. *The Impact of Plague in Tudor and Stuart England.* London: Routledge & Keegan Paul, 1985.

———. "Responses to Plague in Early Modern Europe: The Implications of Public Health." In *In Time of Plague: The History and Social Consequences of Lethal Epidemic Disease,* edited by Arien Mack, 111–32. New York: New York University Press, 1991.

Solomon, Michael. *Fictions of Well-Being: Sickly Readers and Vernacular Medical Writing in Late Medieval and Early Modern Spain.* Philadelphia: University of Pennsylvania Press, 2010.

Stearns, Justin. *Infectious Ideas: Contagion in Premodern Islamic and Christian Thought in the Western Mediterranean.* Baltimore: Johns Hopkins University Press, 2011.

———. "New Directions in the Study of Religious Responses to the Black Death." *History Compass* 7 (2009): 1–13.

Sudhoff, Karl. "Pestschriften aus den ersten 150 Jahren der Epidemie des 'schwarzen Todes.'" *Archiv für Geschichte der Medizin,* 1911–25.

Theilmann, John M., and Frances Cate. "A Plague of Plagues: The Problem of Plague Diagnosis in Medieval England." *Journal of Interdisciplinary History* 37, no. 3 (2007): 371–93.

Thompson, I. A. A., and Bartolomé Yun Casalilla. *The Castilian Crisis of the Seventeenth Century: New Perspectives on the Economic and Social History of Seventeenth-Century Spain.* Cambridge: Cambridge University Press, 1994.

Torre, Esteban. "Las 'Conclusiones' del Doctor Estrada de Madrid, contra los "Avisos Particulares" del Doctor Hidalgo de Agüero, Sevillano." *Asclepio* 30–31 (1978–79): 389–401.

Twigg, Graham. *The Black Death: A Biological Reappraisal.* London: Batsford, 1994.

Vaca de Alfaro, Enrique. *Proposicion Chirvrgica, i censvra ivdiciosa entre las dos vias cvrativas de heridas de cabeça Comun, i Particular, i elecion desta. Con dos epistolas al fin, una de la naturaleza del tumor preternatural, i otra de la patria i origen de Avicena. . . .* Sevilla, 1618.

Valdés, Fernando de. *De la utilidad de la sangria en las viruelas y otras enfermedades de los muchachos.* Sevilla, 1583.

———. *Disputa y averiguaciones de la enfermedad pestilente.* Sevilla, 1600.

Valdivia, Andrés. *Tractado en el qual se explica la essencia y naturaleza de la enfermedad (que llaman landres) que a andado en Sevilla el año de 99 y 600.601.* Sevilla, 1601.

Varela Peris, Fernando. "El papel de la Junta Suprema de Sanidad en la política sanitaria española del siglo XVIII." *Dynamis* 18 (1998): 315–40.

Vassberg, David E. *Land and Society in Golden Age Castile.* Cambridge: Cambridge University Press, 1984.

Velázquez y Sánchez, José. *Anales epidemicos: Reseña historica de las enfermedades contagiosas en Sevilla desde la reconquista cristiana hasta nuestros días (1866).* Reprint, Sevilla: Ayuntamiento de Sevilla, 1996.

Villalba, Joaquin de. *Epidemiologia Española, ó Historia Cronologica de las Pestes, Contagios, Epidemias y Epizootias que han acaecido en España desde la venida de los cartagineses hasta el año 1801.* 2 vols. Madrid, 1803.

Vincent, Bernard. "La peste Atlantica de 1596–1602." *Asclepio* 28 (1976): 5–25.

Viñes Ibarrola, José. *Una epidemica de peste bubónica en el siglo XVI.* Pamplona: Editorial Aramuru, 1947.

Vives, Juan Luis. *De subventione pauperum.* Bruges, 1526.

Wallis, Patrick. "A Dreadful Heritage: Interpreting Epidemic Disease at Eyam, 1666–2000." Working Papers on the Nature of Evidence: How Well Do "Facts" Travel? No. 02/05 (May 2005). http://eprints.lse.ac.uk/22546/1/0205Wallis.pdf.

——. "Plagues, Morality, and the Place of Medicine in Early Modern England." *English Historical Review* 121, no. 490 (2006): 1–24.

Watts, Sheldon. *Epidemics and History: Disease, Power, and Imperialism.* New Haven: Yale University Press, 1997.

Wear, Andrew, Johanna Geyer-Kordesch, and Roger French, eds. *Doctors and Ethics: The Earlier Historical Setting of Professional Ethics.* Amsterdam: Rodopi, 1993.

Williman, Daniel, ed. *The Black Death: The Impact of the Fourteenth-Century Plague.* Binghamton: Center for Medieval and Renaissance Studies, State University of New York at Binghamton, 1982.

Wilson Bowers, Kristy. "Balancing Individual and Communal Needs: Plague and Public Health in Early Modern Seville." *Bulletin of the History of Medicine* 81, no. 2 (2007): 335–58.

——. "Tradition and Innovation in Spanish Medicine: Bartolomé Hidalgo de Agüero and the *Vía Particular.*" *The Sixteenth Century Journal* 41, no. 1 (2010): 29–47.

Wunder, Amanda. "Classical, Christian, and Muslim Remains in the Construction of Imperial Seville (1520–1635)." *Journal of the History of Ideas* 64, no. 2 (2003): 195–212.

Zamudio de Alfaro, Andres. *Orden para la cura y preservacion de las secas y carbuncos. . . .* Madrid, 1599.

——. *Orden para la cura y preservacion de la viruelas.* Madrid, 1579.

——. *Tractado de peste.* Sevilla, 1569.

Ziegler, Philip. *The Black Death.* New York: John Day, 1969.

Index

Printed in the USA
CPSIA information can be obtained
at www.ICGtesting.com
LVHW042038181223
766775LV00004B/103